WISDOM OF THE SENSES

OTHER WORKS
BY JOHN HERLIHY

Near and Distant Horizons: In Search of the
Primary Sources of Knowledge

Journeys With Soul:
Adventures & Cures That Came True

Wisdom's Journey: Living the Spirit of Islam
in the Modern World

Borderlands of the Spirit: Reflections on a
Sacred Science of Mind

The Essential René Guénon: Metaphysics, Tradition,
and the Crisis of Modernity

Modern Man at the Crossroads: The Encounter of
Modern Science & Traditional Knowledge

The Seeker and the Way: Reflections of a Muslim Convert

Veils and Keys: Contemporary Reflections
on Traditional Islamic Themes

JOHN HERLIHY

WISDOM
OF
THE SENSES

THE UNTOLD STORY
OF THEIR INNER LIFE

∾

SOPHIA PERENNIS

SAN RAFAEL, CA

First published in the USA
by Sophia Perennis
© John Herlihy 2010

Series editor: James R. Wetmore

For information, address:
Sophia Perennis, P.O. Box 151011
San Rafael, CA 94915
sophiaperennis.com

Library of Congress Cataloging-in-Publication Data

Herlihy, John.
Wisdom of the senses : the untold story
of their inner life / John Herlihy.
p. cm.
ISBN 978-1-59731-127-4 (pbk.: alk. paper)
1. Psychology, Religious. 2. Senses and sensation—Religious
aspects. 3. Wisdom. 4. Spirituality. I. Title.
BL53.H415 2010
200.1'9—dc22   2010050701

CONTENTS

PREFACE

The Untold Story

Ancient mysteries continue to haunt the psyche of the modern mentality with their inscrutable questions. In spite of the advanced technologies modern science has made available to the general public that virtually set the pace and define today's culture and civilization, we have yet to crack the code that will lead us beyond the horizon of our time. Although scientists have explored deep down into the unpredictable laws of the quantum world in our search for the building blocks of matter hoping to find in the words of Stephen Hawkins "a unified theory of everything", people today still have no clear answers they can believe with any certainty to give definition and shape to their earthly lives. We have relied on the human mind and its faculty of reason to think our way through the labyrinth of speculation and doubt that marks the centerpiece of the modern secular worldview. Similarly, the premier instruments of investigation supporting the scientific method are none other than the five senses that on their own, or in tandem with the recently developed rarefied pieces of scientific equipment that attempt to document at the quantum level and through empirical evidence the true nature of reality.[1] In the end, we still rely on seeing, hearing, smelling, tasting, and touching in order to declare what we believe to be an objective reality.

This work was originally intended to make up a brief little book. After all, how much can you say about the five senses or the inscrutable sixth sense that we no longer believe in. It is true that the five senses make demands on our bodies without ever giving up their

---

1. Instruments such as the telescopes in deep space or the supercollider that records the activity of the quantum world onto electro-magnetic tape.

insatiable desire. This in itself is a commentary on their use and function that fairly summarizes the intense nature of their demands on the body. In addition, the mysterious "ghost" of the senses keeps us guessing about whether the objectivity they offer the modern mentality is truly convincing. There is no denying that the demands of the senses ride us as though they were riding an invisible tiger, leaving behind in their wake an echo of disenchantment that keeps us wondering whether we are using these instruments of knowledge and perception to full advantage. We see, hear, smell, taste and touch the world; but for all of their demands, the senses never bring the satisfaction their experiences promise. They are the portals of pleasure as well as the instruments of verification of the physical reality; but where is the resolution to their promise of certitude and where is the satisfaction that their desires foreshadow?

This effort is intended for a special audience. After all, the preface endeavors to address the needs of those who might be inclined to pick up this book in a bookstore and give it two minutes of their attention before setting it back down again and passing on. Publishers, distributors and agents of all kinds tell us that the title is crucial and the effect on the mind of a potential reader can make or break a good book in the five seconds it takes for the title's import to register as worthy of further attention. The two key words of the title, of course, are wisdom and senses. There is strangeness to their juxtaposition and intimacy in their close proximity. We do not normally think of the senses as wise, even if we appreciate their benefits and pursue their promises with devotion and relentless attention to detail. We may use the senses as instruments of verification for our scientific experiments and call upon the mystique of their supposed objectivity to identify once and for all the true nature, not only of the physical world, but also by some strange analogy, the universal reality. However, we do not usually call the senses wise. Wisdom is for saints and Tibetan lamas and Indian gurus. The wisdom generated by the senses is knowledge turned inside out, exposing the eternal verities in the clear light of an eternal day, and not the routine and calculated facts that we encounter in the everyday world, much less the desires the senses serve that drag us deeper down into the world of the flesh.

This work is intended to explore the full dimensions of the five senses as portals and passageways into the interior of ourselves as a prelude to rising above ourselves in surrender and unity with God. Let us explore the vision of seeing by looking with both eyes upon the signs and symbols of the Creator Who has given us the gift of sight. Let us listen to the revelatory sounds that abound within nature and that have descended in the form of verses of the Holy Book, the Quran. The celebrated Islamic poet and mystic Rumi writes: "Birds' voices and the grove's moody colors offer immortality when we enter the garden, you and I." Let us taste the nutritional wonders of the created universe in remembrance of the One who has fashioned all created things from His own Hand according to the truth of their true nature. Let us smell the essence of things in light of their truth and remember the blessing of the paradise in which all earthly smells are but a pale reflection. Let us feel the texture and grain of things with our fingers, slowly and softly experiencing the touch and feel of the wondrous reality of this world as prelude and first step to experiencing the truth of some higher realm of experience. Let us walk toward the One Who has given us a body that stands upon feet that can make their way. According to Rumi, "Your head is but a lamp with six wicks: Without that spark, would any remain alight?"[2] Indeed, what is the spark that will illuminate the six wicks of our senses? What will illuminate the light of the mind if there is no luminous source? Where is the spark the will ignite the smouldering embers of a darkened heart?

This modest book is intended to expose the mystery of the sixth sense and the intuitive knowledge whose perception can take us by the hand and lead us out of ourselves. The sixth sense is the apex and summit of the other five senses. When the Quran says: Vision grasps Him not, but He grasps all vision" (6:103), we understand the reference to vision as the Supreme Intellect of which the human intellect is a pale but certain reflection. The sixth sense is to the mind what the other five senses are to the body, namely a portal of perception to the mystery of the Unseen and the knowledge of God

2. Mevlana Jalaluddin Rumi, *Rumi's Divan of Shems of Tabriz: Selected Odes* (Rockport, MA: Element, 1997) p. 137.

that would otherwise be unknown to the human mind. If there is a physical counterpart to intuition, it would be the heart which is actually the seat of the intelligence in the Islamic tradition. Once again, Rumi writes: "Those with mirror-like hearts do not depend on fragrance and color: they behold Beauty in the moment. They've cracked open the shell of knowledge and raised the banner of the eye of certainty. Thought is gone in a flash of light."[3]

There must be more to the five senses than insatiable desire or a pseudo objectivity that explains away universal reality by reducing it to the sub-atomic world of atoms and molecules. In the profound darkness of the night, the time when people perennially turn inward in search of something more than the surface experience on offer to the senses during the daytime, myths give rise to meaning and legends are born that people can listen to, if they have sense enough to recognize the benefit of silence and see darkness as an opportunity for inner light. In the evening, sit under the stars and see what the universe has to offer. The stillness of the night is full of the most varied voices, sounds and whispers, if the astute mind chooses to listen, and the black velvet of the night sky is perforated by specks of light as though the light of some eternal universe were hidden behind its plate of darkness. In truth, the distant stars are but elegant fire flies that speckle the night with their phosphorescent beauty. The darkness itself contains sights and smells that come from everywhere to assault the senses with their mystery and their promise, from behind the tree, from under the ground, from the depths of the dark night. During the daytime, the senses take up the cup of sweet pleasure and drain it dry. They smell the aromatic odors of the world; they delight in the provocative visions the natural world has on offer; they taste the nectar of every edible vegetable and fruit; but behind the formal structure of eyes, ears, nose, mouth, and skin lies a frightening array of sensations in the form of visions, silences, smells and experiences of taste and touch that have the power to rock our inner worlds with the secrets they contain and the wisdom they reveal.

3. *The Inner Journey: Views from the Islamic Tradition*, ed. William C. Chittick (Sandpoint, ID: Morning Light Press, 2007), p. 202.

To open your mind and heart to the true messages of the senses is to cross a mythic threshold in order to stand on the front line of spiritual experience. Nothing prevents the natural interaction of the physical world with the higher world of the spirit. There are no compromises, no stages of development, no pretending. There is only the perennial battle to lift the veil that separates us from the direct vision of the Divinity, to see the invisible, to hear the inaudible, to taste the intuitions of the mind with their direct experience of the supernatural and to bask in the feelings of certitude that shower upon the soul that is receptive to the influences of the spirit. The on-going battle of the soul that Islam proclaims as the ultimate challenge of the human condition takes place first and foremost within the life of the senses, as knowledge of the senses becomes manifest as wisdom with the power to transform the life experience into a journey toward transcendence of the human condition. The richness and diversity of the world is not experienced in purely physical, palpable, tangible and visible forms, but in view of its symbolic significance that all traditional people imparted to every river, mountain and star.

We go through life witnessing the world through the blessing of sight and we take wing and fly toward the vision of the Divinity witnessed through the "eye" of the heart. We listen to the sound vibrations of every created thing and incorporate their rhythms into the harmony of our waking moments, enriched by the sound of the cricket and the fluttering of the moth, enchanted by the cry of the peacock and enthralled by the thunder and lightning of heaven. We make our way through the world smelling the essence of things from the clove of garlic to lilies in a pond and thus become privy through aromatic smells to the very essence and soul of an object. We occupy our days with the requirements of eating and drinking to sustain the physical body, but even the mundane moments of our everyday life can take on the magic and mystery of some untold secret if we taste the world through the intuitions the mind makes available to us.

In addition, the preface is intended to give a taste, for want of a better word, of what is to come within the main body of the work. Like a drop of honey, the reader can sample the essence of the book in terms of content and style in a few concise words without being overwhelmed by the totality of the message. Throughout this work, we reflect upon and explore the possibilities inherent in the sentential experiences of the five senses, partly because we hope to expose the myth that the senses exist only to serve our human, physical needs and are only the expression of our insatiable desire for satisfaction of the body, and partly to rekindle the wisdom and love of God in counterpoint to the knowledge and desire imparted by the attractions of only "this world". The superficial goal of the senses is to love and embrace the pleasures of this world. The more we embrace that which the world has to offer, the more we become entrenched in its superficial delights, merely stoking the flames of desire and leaving behind the cold embers of dissatisfaction. The inner goal of the senses is to love and embrace the Beloved as the object of our truest desire. The more we embrace that which God has on offer for us, the more we transcend the world and leave it behind, creating a burning within the heart that never dies, but rather becomes a cooling flame and a fireless heat, producing the alchemy of the soul as the singular expression, not of the individual, but of the Divinity. In a famous *hadith qudsi* that actually represents the words of God, the Prophet said: "My servant never ceases approaching Me through voluntary works until I love him. Then, when I love him, I am the hearing through which he hears, the seeing through which he sees, the hand through which he grasps, and the feet through which he walks."

It is incredible to think that we rely on the senses in so many ways without ever tapping their true reserves and without ever realizing their full capacity to reveal the inside story of our experience of the world. We eat, drink, smell the flowers and reach out to others without ever waking up to the secret import of these experiences and their effect on psyche and soul. We listen to music, for example, and what do we hear but pleasant melodies that make us smile or move us to their rhythm and beat; but the act of creative love generated by the creation of a beautiful and moving melody and the manner in which the music transports us to other realms are soon forgotten, if never fully realized. We live in the age of communication and are supposed to appreciate the power of words and their ability to

communicate meaning and message; but the power of sound to reflect sacred harmonies and to transport us through the resonance
and vibratory qualities of sacred revelation, for example, are lost on
our busy mentalities. We hear the sound; but we are not truly listening to the music. Just as the inner faculties of reason, intelligence,
heart knowledge, consciousness, spiritual imagination and sacred
instinct, all lead us out of ourselves and make transcendence of the
human condition possible, so also the five senses and the comple-
mentary sixth sense are sentential instruments of knowledge and
perception that we need to more fully explore and experience, if we
ever wish to understand the universal mystery that underscores all
existence. We must recognize this mystery as a fundamental truth of
our existential reality, if we are ever to achieve the knowledge of the
true reality that all men, scientists included, unequivocally profess
to be the ultimate goal of the modern, thinking individual.

Imagine the finger of God upon our sense of touch, the hand of
God upon our hands. We could do no wrong and everything we
might accomplish with our hands would contain the signature of
the Divinity. Imagine seeing and smelling the world through God's
eyes and all on behalf of a mutual love between the Divine and the
human with which nothing can compare. Imagine the presence of
the Divinity taking up residence within the human heart in fulfilment of the promise that the human body is the temple of the spirit
and that "the Kingdom of God is within you.", as we learn from the
New Testament. The Quran tells us explicitly that "God is with you
wherever you are" (57:4) and perhaps a little more ominously that
"Allah comes between man and his own heart." (8:24) There is perhaps no limit to what humans can accomplish, provided our works
are measured against the relationship we have with God. The
human journey can become a spiritual adventure without taking
leave of the reality of this world, by understanding the human
senses and the ubiquitous sixth sense, not as instruments to verify
the objectivity of the physical world, but rather as portals to a
higher world of understanding that attempts to describe the presence of God in the world as well as in the human heart.

We are the bell that when struck resounds with the harmonies of
a true reality that binds us together into a seamless whole. We are

the reed flute that, when blown upon by the "breath of the Compassionate", creates the voice and the soul of the virtuous man. When the human being plays its own delicate instrument and becomes its own reed flute, the sentient portals of the body, like the apertures of the flute, become capable of whispering the resolution of God's mysteries. The senses have a story to tell and it will be told. They have a music to play whose reverberations will echo across the wide open spaces of a life well lived. They have a song to sing and it will be sung, as long as the earth abides and humanity lives on to experience and absorb the wise messages the senses have to offer.

> *Now I will tell you without speech and with constant renewal*
> *The ancient mysteries: Listen!*
> (Rumi, Mathnawi III 4684)

1

THE SECRET
LIFE OF THE SENSES

Unless the eye catch fire
The God will not be seen.
Unless the ear catch fire
The God will not be heard
Unless the tongue catch fire
The God will not be named
Unless the heart catch fire
The God will not be loved
Unless the mind catch fire
The God will not be known.[1]

Strange as it may seem, a complete narrative of the five senses is a story that has yet to be fully told. We rely on our senses as the anchors of sentience in order to perceive and understand the world we inhabit. We use our senses as vehicles of pleasure to heighten, if not our complete happiness, then at least our random and nominal enjoyment of the world. They raise us up to the heavens where eagles soar and streaks of lightning move like jagged arrows across the heavens. They cast us down with their insatiable desires into the deepest subterranean well where the sky becomes a reflection of distant light and dreams of soaring mountain peaks are forgotten. Scientists throughout history have relied on the senses as the instruments of knowing and perception, as well as the filter through which the world around us can be objectified as a categorical truth as well as an existential reality. Because of the senses, we have the

1. Quoted from Theodore Roszak, *Where the Wasteland Ends* (New York, NY: Doubleday & Company, Inc., 1972), p. 296–297.

ability to know, experience, and respond to the world around us in order to take part in the life it has to offer. We take in, internalize, and become a true reflection of the mysterious world we encounter, thanks to the immediacy of the senses. One question remains, however, that disturbs the serenity of our initial inquiry: Is that enough? Is it enough that we can meet the world on our own terms with these unique instruments of perception, anchors as it were that can ground us in the reality of "this world"? Hopefully, it is a question worth pursuing throughout the course of this book, one that may reveal an unexpected and surprising outcome.

Just as the four elements of earth, air, fire, and water represent the *materia prima* of the natural order, these solid, aerial, fiery, and fluid modes of manifestation have communicated their sacred quality to the five senses down through history, senses that in themselves also partake of a sacred and inner quality that transcends their literal and outward experience. Throughout the millennia, humanity has relied on the open receptivity of the five senses to capture the essential form of an object and in so doing create the sense—for want of a better word—of the reality of a thing as the initial step in the understanding of the reality of the world and the surrounding universe beyond that world. The five senses are the first tier of experience in a range of faculties and modes of perception that we have available to us in what amounts to a great adventure in pursuit of an understanding of the reality we live in without knowing the full extent of its true meaning and significance.

Beyond the five senses there lies a number of human faculties including intuition, intelligence, reason, imagination, and the holy sentiments that help us make our way through a labyrinth of mystery that confronts us in this world. In addition, the higher faculties support the attitude of faith and the force field of the human will to accept the higher knowledge of a traditional worldview to embrace and believe in, followed by the actions, disciplines and good works that make up the human manifestation in this world of these universal principles. None of the apertures of perception and experience can have any true value without the opening of the heart, which in a number of traditions, including the Religion of Islam, is the "seat of the intelligence" as well as the repository of the higher human sentiments. In other words, what we see, hear, smell, taste and feel through the body enters by way of the five senses, passes through the filter of the mind, explores the enlivening realm of the sacred human emotions, only to find their true place within the consciousness of humanity through the portal of the heart which is not contained within space, but that has space enough to contain the mystery of all that we see, hear, smell, taste and touch.

In the wake of an epic and perennial struggle to differentiate a true understanding of the role of both matter and spirit in resolving the mystery of human identify in relation to the Face (*al-wajh*) of the Supreme Being, we have brought the search for the true nature of reality during the post-modern era to its logical conclusion with the scientific worldview in which matter serves as the ultimate reality, and anything that does not abide by our three dimensional world and the input of our five senses simply does not exist. Of course, the ancients thought otherwise and took inspiration from the words of Christ when he is reported to have said: "I shall give you what no eye has seen and what no ear has heard and what no hand has touched and what has never occurred to the human mind."[2] People who partook of a more traditional environment knew and appreciated that the convention of form is transcended by the largesse of spirit, just as the flicker of a flame gives way to the incandescence of light. The visionary impulses of their mentality laid claim to a third eye, fifth dimension and sixth sense whose inner door opened onto the open skies of an invisible, indeed a spiritual world, much like air and breath are the vital components of life itself, that lies beyond the dimension of sight, that ultimately comes to a pinnacle as a single, universal reality known throughout the ages as the Transcendent, the Absolute, the Beneficent whose Spirit "hovers over the waters", but that is universally understood by the name God, the Supreme Being. As quoted in the epigraph at the beginning of this chapter, unless the five physical senses and various human faculties[3] "catch

2. "Eye hath not seen nor ear heard, nor hath it entered into the heart of man." (1 Corinthians 2:9)

3. In Sanskrit, *vijñāna*, or the eight consciousnesses, all sentient beings possess: sight, hearing, smell, taste, touch, and three different operations of the mind.

fire", the Transcendent Reality cannot be experienced and the Presence of God cannot be known. All else becomes as a fireless smoke amid the smoldering ruins of our human spiritual aspirations.

The soul is never satisfied until it uncovers the mystery contained within forms and it will never be truly content until it finds its final abode in the spirit that substantiates and ultimately transcends all natural forms. In terms of sheer functionality, the import and significance of the senses play a major role in experiencing the world of forms. Beyond the literal and formal input of the senses lies the wisdom of their true meaning. The five senses dutifully record what they see, hear, smell, taste and touch; but beyond their formal and functional aspect lies a visionary wisdom that intuits the inner meaning of things, that listens to the echo of a universal revelation that comes down to humanity in a variety of forms through nature, messengers and scriptures. The senses arouse memories and histories and dreams of a deeper truth than the physical forms that on their own give lie to a higher essence contained in the form. When we see the early morning rooster, we await the sound of its awakening call; when we see the owl perched on a tree limb at night, we imagine its eerie hoot sounding its audible waves through the stillness of the pines.

> *Amidst the notes*
> *Of my koto is another*
> *Deep mysterious tone,*
> *A sound that comes from*
> *Within my own breast.*[4]

However, what the inner spirit yearns for, and therefore relies on the inner nature of the senses to proclaim, is to listen to the cock when it has not yet uttered its cry, to feel the reverberations of a bell before it has been struck, or to intuit the unique wisdom of the owl's hoot without actually listening to the sound.

---

4. Yosano Akiko, *One Hundred More Poems from the Japanese,* translated by Kenneth Rexroth (New York, 1974), quoted from *Music in the Sky,* ed. by Patrick Laude & Barry McDonald (Bloomington: IN: World Wisdom Books, 2004).

Every human sense contains a deep well of knowledge and insight that reveals to the unsuspecting mind what lies beyond the physicality of the world. This knowledge through forms and images and sounds create impressions of what lies within an experience and emerges upon a plane of higher consciousness for what lies beyond the horizon of the known world. Enclosed within all the sensations that cannot be verified, the thoughts that cannot be resolved, and the dreams that cannot come true, lies the spirit of an ancient, primordial reality that is never wrong and can never fade away. From these outermost instruments of human perception flow rarefied knowledge and sensory experience that sink down into the innermost depths of our nature where their impressions and insights nurture and grow until we awaken toward a feeling of mystery as a prelude to a higher consciousness of truth, just as surely as we awaken to the new day with the sweet sound of the birds and the gentle patter of rain. What the inner aspect of the senses conveys is not knowledge or wisdom precisely and is almost impossible to categorize. Buried deep within the human being lies an inmost presence, a witness if you will, that knows everything that needs to be known, in a place where mystery and intuition unite to give birth to an instinctive faith in the Unseen; but how this primordial presence is stirred to consciousness to give shape to a disciplined mind and a devotional heart requires great discipline in the appreciation and use of the human senses.

We have all experienced the mystery of the senses without coming to terms with their inner power and wisdom, inspiring William Blake to remark, "A fool sees not the same tree that a wise man sees." As compensation for their loss, the blind man may see an inner light that leads to a road seldom traveled; the deaf man hears the vibratory frequencies that form the texture of a universe that escapes ordinary, human ears; but leads him effectively to some unexpected destination. Animals use the power of scent as a source of knowledge and guidance, while many a simple smell, from the perfume of flowers to the smoke of burning autumn leaves, can arouse an evocation to memory and recreate the heart of an experience that we hold dear. What some people see as the curtain of night appears to others as a milky way of stars. We listen and see; but we do not hear

the voice of lightning, trace the music that lies behind the movement of the eyes, or smell the sweet fragrance of the spoken word.
The glow of a color or the fragrance of a scent can never come of
their own power; but are instead the reflection of some greater miracle. When we say that we see the light and hear the music, language
itself fails, especially when it comes to conveying the inner meaning
of an experience. We could just as easily refer to the fragrance of the
color and the glow of the scent to arrive at a meaning that conveys
its true miracle, well beyond the lateral thinking of the mind. When
we refer to the music of light or the vision of sound, are we speaking
in meaningless terms or are we perhaps arriving through another
door to the inner meaning of an experience that cannot be contained through the literal use of words; but that transmits an alternative meaning through the linguistic magic of suggestion and
innuendo. To cite a poem of Daito, a Japanese poet who lived from
1282–1337:

> *When one sees with ears*
> *And hears with eyes,*
> *One cherishes no doubts.*
> *How naturally the raindrops*
> *Fall from the leaves!*[5]

Isn't sound itself the absence of silence; while silence constitutes
the absence of sound, acting as if the sheer power of the void were
listening from some region beyond the auricular dimension altogether. There is a curious interpenetration when the eternal void of
soundlessness actually penetrates the world of sound with its ethereal and everlasting quality of suggestivity and potential; while the
sound in its living reality inspires the eternal soundlessness that is
the hallmark of inner peace. A flowered landscape is as beautiful as
the golden embroidery of a silken brocade and has a life of
unknown mystery that is proclaimed by its existence; but it is the
singing of the birds and the buzzing of the bees that would bring
this portrait to life with the promise of an eternal soundlessness that

---

5. Quoted in *The Buddha Eye: An Anthology of the Kyoto School and Its Contem-
poraries*, ed. Frederick Frank (Bloomington, IN: World Wisdom Books, 2004), p. 7.

lies with latent power beyond the utterance of sound, wrapped and unfurled within the tapestry of the natural order.

There is a power to the senses that calls to mind the birth of a river in the appearance of a bubbling stream or that witnesses the design of a flower in the emerging rose bud. When we see the mountains, do we ask ourselves when they were laid upon the earth or what they mean in terms of stability and strength; when we hear the roar of the oceans or the howl of the wind, do we wonder about the sacred voice behind the creation of these things; when we witness the night sky, do we wonder who has scattered those distant stars across the field of night like diamonds on black velvet and do we witness the sky-blue vault of the heavens as the formless infinitude that it really is? We can easily be deceived by the magic of a name and the suggestion of its meaning, but we can never touch the inner substance of a fact without moving beyond the outer experience of the senses.

> *To listen to the music of the Sky;*
> *And then to realize: the Song was I.*[6]

Such is the mystery and the wisdom embodied within the physical world of the senses that the messages they convey allow us "one foot in Eden", according to John Muir and from that vantage point give us insight from the "other land" into the world of time, of history, and of the sensory input of "this world". We only begin to awaken to this reality when we realize that the material world, the world of space and time as it appears to our outer senses, is nothing but a sign and symbol of the mysterious spirit that transcends these wayward phenomena.

∼

Before we embark on a voyage into the unknown world of the inner life of the senses, we need to consider briefly what the outer senses have to offer us and the role they have been set to play in negotiating our way within the human kingdom that we inhabit. In today's

6. "The Song", Frithjof Schuon, *Road to the Heart*, (Bloomington, IN: World Wisdom Books, 1995).

world, science strives for objectivity through the use of the five outer[7] senses. We are able to verify to the satisfaction of the rational mind what the senses tell us. What we cannot verify directly, we then verify indirectly through rarefied technologies that record activity of the atomic and quantum worlds when the direct vision of the eyes fails to witness and record what takes place at the sub-atomic level As such, scientists boast that the pursuits and discoveries of modern science make the full disclosure of the physical reality well within our reach, either through the instruments of the senses or through the pursuit of an instrumental science that has prodigiously extended its grasp over physical reality.

Today's scientific worldview can now boast that having been blind for millennia, we can now see the invisible—literally—with the naked eye (with the aid of rarefied instruments of course, amounting to an indirect literal viewing at best). We have learned, for example, that visible light is not the only illuminating energy within the universe. It is actually an infinitesimal spec of electro-magnetic radiation comprising wave lengths of 400 to 700 nanometers (billionths of a meter), creating radiation that rains continuously down upon our bodies. Before modern-day instruments developed the capacity to measure such activity, we were oblivious to its existence. When we were once deaf; now everything is available to our ears through the use of rarefied instruments that not only imitate, but actually mock the skills of the natural senses. Humans have a natural auditory range from 20 to 20,000 Hz per second. Now we know that flying bats broadcast ultrasonic pulses into the night air above that range and listen for echoes to locate moths and other insects on the wing. Before the 1950s, zoologists were unaware of this nocturnal contest, Today, with specially attuned receivers, transformers and night-time photography, they can follow every squeak and aerial "bat and mouse" performance

---

7. In making distinctions through this chapter between outer and inner senses, we wish to explore and highlight the distinction that needs to be made between the capacity of the senses to explore, measure and document the world on the one hand, as well as their innate ability to awaken the mind, heart and soul to higher level of perception and experience.

between predator and prey, all at auditory ranges beyond the reach of humans.

The descent into *minutissima* in the search for the ultimate building blocks seems to be the driving motivation, some people might call it mania, of modern science in the attempts of its practitioners to unveil and identify a complete and definitive theory of knowledge that would lay to rest once and for all any alternative claims to the true nature of reality, such as those that the traditional worldview sets forth. This search for the ultimate particle in quantum physics has been aided through steady advances in the resolving power of microscopes, in response to the ultimate human craving to see all of reality with the human eye. The most powerful modern instruments developed in the 1980s are the scanning-tunneling microscope and the atomic force microscope which provide an almost literal view of atoms bonded into molecules and the DNA double helix. Atomic-level imaging is the end product of three centuries of technological innovation in search of direct observation with the "unaided eye", although in this case it is the "aided eye" that makes these technically miraculous discoveries. Microscopy began with the primitive optical instruments of Anton van Leeuwenhoek, which in the late 1600s revealed bacteria and other objects a hundred times smaller than the resolution of the human eye. It has arrived at methods for showing objects a million times smaller, resulting now in the fast developing science of nanotechnology.

As a result, the haphazard, sensory capacity of instruments that has led to the classification of data and their interpretation by theory, when taken together, extend beyond belief the rational processing of sensory experience enhanced by instrumentation. This worked well enough in the favor of scientists until they discovered that solid matter, the very ground upon which the scientific enterprise stands and the foundation that bears the weight of the entire fabric of modern science, is actually nothing more than empty space. The solidity of iron is actually 99.9999999999 percent vacuous space strangely enough, made to feel solid by ethereal force fields that have no material reality. Quantum physics has now revealed that what we perceive as a particle may also be a wave and vise versa, amounting to the conjecture that, on the physical plane, there is no fixed or tangible reality at all, a truth casting its pale light onto the principles of transcendence that the religions have proclaimed all along.

Let us consider, for example, the sound of music. The waves of sound enter the eardrum in a beautifully complex path, only to become electrical pulses that are chemically stored in the cortex of the brain. But how do we hear the sound and how does its implicit beauty become apparent and appreciated? Where is the vision, sound or smell of the senses once it reaches the mind, much less the heart? Just which of those formerly inert atoms of carbon, hydrogen, nitrogen, oxygen, and so on in my head have become so clever that they can produce a thought or reconstitute an image or sound? How sense data are recalled and replayed into sentience remains an enigmatic mystery to modern science without an impending solution at hand. We are still in search of the passageways that lead from the brain to the mind and eventually flow into the ocean of consciousness that we take for granted as an inevitable gift of life, even though we cannot put our finger on it or give its workings a name.

We live within a certain frame of reference and are subject to the contingencies of the natural order; but "when we observe the sentient wisdom of life emerging from the physical structures replete within the natural order, we are witnessing the emergence of a parameter not evident in those structures."[8] We know that atoms join together to form a brain that generate neural impulses of a thought within a mind that ultimately are translated into well constructed thoughts and desires. What, however, is the true relationship between a desire and the senses that crave physical satisfaction? There is a growing certainty among some of today's scientists that there are even dimensions in our universe that we cannot sense, regardless of how clever and precise our instrumentation may eventually become. We see the results of experiments; but we can't follow the reactions that lead to those results because physics actually operates within certain insensible dimensions that we cannot calculate or measure, even with precise instruments. The philosopher

8. Gerald L. Schroeder, *The Hidden Face of God* (New York, NY: The Free Press, 2001), p. 15.

Moses Maimonides, in his famous book appropriately entitled *The Guide of the Perplexed* clearly stated his position over 800 years ago: "We must form a conception of the existence of the Creator according to our capacities, that is, we must have a knowledge of metaphysics (the science of God) which can only be acquired after the study of physics (the science of nature); for the science of physics is closely connected with metaphysics and must even precede it in the course of studies."[9] Modern physics has now entered the metaphysical, the realm beyond the physically perceivable, in the fullest sense of that word.

There is a side of reality that does not fit into the physical universe as we know and experience it in our everyday lives; but do we allow our senses to perceive in our minds and record in our hearts the sacred messages they convey? Perhaps this is the meaning behind the metacosmic symbol of the universe itself, that through the course of its fathomless depths lies a message of eternity and infinity. If anything around us is truly marked with the seal of universality, it is the universe itself that surrounds us, penetrates us and reflects what we are made of. Today scientists marvel in their discoveries of black holes and speculate in wonder about parallel universes; quantum physicists have explored deep down into the heart of the nuclear world only to find the conundrum of the particle and the wave that dazzles us with its enigmatic quality and the hazy indeterminism of the quantum world, but leaves us bereft of a comprehensible meaning and significance beyond a curious hinting at freedom and creativity, leaving the mass population awash in a flood of facts and figures that have no inner import beyond the raw information they convey.

Even the act of sense perception, the very act upon which all our knowledge is supposed to be based during this modern and so called enlightened era of techno-discovery, has become incomprehensible to us, draining away the mystery from the universe and leaving us wandering in a labyrinth of speculative, analogical knowledge masquerading in the guise of true knowledge. We have lost the child that

9. Quoted in *The Hidden Face of God*, Gerald L. Schroeder (NY, New York: The New Free Press, 2001), pp. 23–24.

once existed within ourselves whose sense of intuition remained simple and pure until such time that it became corrupted by the experience of our modern world and its forms of enlightenment. The child lives in a world of perpetual wonder; every experience is new and enchanting, creating an exultation of innocent spirit whose simple, uncluttered mind turns every symbolic form of nature into a poetic metaphor. The twittering of birds is a cause for joy; dust particles sparkling in a ray of light invite curiosity and a smile. The natural world is sharpened by the attention and perspicacity of seeing, hearing and smelling as if for the first time. If only we could have retained the natural force of those infant first experiences, for they lead to discrimination, awakening and the memory of what once was "in the beginning", *in illo tempore*. If we attempt to contemplate the inner meaning that lies beyond the outer form of every created thing, then we would be endowed with the sacred power of the owl, Athena's bird resting in the sacred olive tree, who could "see in the night" and utters the distinctive hoot that becomes for all to hear an echo of some deeper experience of wonder.

Beyond the physical data gathered by the outer senses we perceive nothing; our first premises do not permit the search and exploration of mystery, when all the while the mystery is there to be experienced and surprisingly simple to behold once the veil of "this world" has been lifted from our physical eyes. Seeing, hearing and the like— these miraculous prodigies of witnessing and perception—are God-given gifts in a God-created world, consisting of the five senses, a mind to process what the senses experience, and a heart to seal their knowledge and insight as a realized intuition and an internalized perception. We must learn to see with the inner eye, to listen to the harmonies that emerge from the forms of nature, to smell the unique perfume that characterizes the essence of every created thing, to taste and ultimately feel with the body, mind, and heart the truth of the world, by involving the whole person, including the body, mind, heart and soul. Nature speaks not of herself but of her Maker. "Heaven and Earth are full of thy glory" the Quran proclaims. Qualitative or spiritual elements are not subject to the verification of the senses; no amount of experimental research can either prove or disprove their presence in the physical world.

Nature does not withhold the glories of its miraculous vistas from my expectant senses; but are the five delicate instruments of perception sufficiently tuned to receive these incredible images with intelligence and grace? The night sky is the perennial field of optical wonders and a realm of discovery for the fertile imagination, even though most of us walk around with our eyes to the ground as half of our universe passes us by unnoticed. I have written elsewhere that while walking alone in the desert late one afternoon, I suddenly had the distinct impression that my surroundings had become the venue of some vast infinity. It was as though "I had fallen through a crack in the universe to find that the mystery of life was suddenly exposed to the crude witnessing of my sense of sight. Something within me had also broken open to allow the in-pouring of a knowledge that transcended the input of the senses. Overhead the night sky was rippling with stars, like diamond chips against black velvet, highlighting in their infinitesimality the blackness of the heavens and sending their infinite specks of light across millions of light years, to reach my curious eye and enter my mind in order to create a profound sense of wonder and awe that complemented the cloud of descending dusk that cast shadows across the land."[10]

The heavenly night sky provides a roaming ground for the angels and has been called by St. Augustine the "city of God", but to move freely within its symbolic ambiance, we must cultivate our senses, and not the least our sense of wonder through the five physical instruments available to us. Such sights as the night sky, such smells as the odor of the rose, and such flavors as the nectar of honey are the building blocks that nature provides for us to construct our inner being and give the soul its true aura and poignancy. It may take the effort of a lifetime; but it is worth distinguishing ourselves from the buzzing and twittering and gurgling confusion of the world. It is through the five senses that the soul can float in and out from the self to the world and back again, touching the world with its own poignancy and being touch in return by the wonders of the natural order. Like water, the soul takes in all impressions and

10. *Wisdom's Journey: Living the Spirit of Islam in the Modern World* (Bloomington, IN: World Wisdom Books, 2009) p. 74.

follows all forms before giving itself back out into the world, all the while remaining true to its undivided essence. "The soul of man resembles water," wrote Goethe[11], thereby reiterating an image that occurs in the Scriptures of both Near and Far East. The soul resembles water, just as the Spirit is spoken of with reference to wind or air. Perhaps this explains the great calming effect the soul has on individuals when they gaze upon the waters of the great oceans and rivers of the world. The Quran echoes the symbolic value of water as the essential, primordial source of the creation with the words: "We have created every living thing from water." (21:30)

In today's world, the primary aim of individuals is to satiate the senses, while in the traditional world, their primary purpose is to reveal the essence behind the physical forms and convey to the human sensibility the true messages that substantiate those outer forms. What allows the input of the senses to become a refined experience with purpose and devotion is their effective use and application through acts of spiritual discipline and discovery amounting to a mastery over the impulses of the senses in order to reveal their inner messages, transforming the sense of sight into a sense of inner vision, the sense of hearing into a sense of the sacred vibration that accompanies the sound of every created form, the innate sense of smell that identifies the inner essence of a thing through the expression of its unique odor. Mastery over the outer senses, with their analytical and discursive tendencies, leads to the revelation of the inner spiritual senses, and their immediate awakening to a higher knowledge and experience than could not otherwise be known by the human mind on its own in a world of purely physical sensations.

Discipline of the eyes requires a turning away from the impurities of the world of thought and aspiration, clouding the vision of our hopes and dreams with mundane desires that will drag us through the underbelly of the world of forms. The Islamic fast during the holy month of Ramadhan is not just refraining from food and drink

---

11. *The Origins of European Thought: About the Body, the Mind, the Soul, the World, Time, and Fate* (Cambridge: Cambridge University Press, 2nd Rev. Edition, 1988) p. 209.

as a rigorous discipline of the body, but also serves as a rigorous inner discipline requiring will power over the demanding forces of the senses of seeing, hearing, and tasting and a deliberate effort at mastery of their pernicious and unending demands. In the Chinese spiritual tradition, fasting also had both an outer and inner aspect that created a holistic effect on the body. "Can you tell me the way?" one of his companions asked the famous Chinese sage. "Fast," Confucius replied, "and I will tell you the way." The follower said: "I have not tasted wine or meat for several months. Is this not enough of a fast?" "It is merely liturgical fast," said Confucius, "but not the fast of mind." "What is the fast of mind?" asked Yen Jui, and Confucius answered: "Maintain the unity of your will. Cease to listen with the ear, but listen with the mind. Cease to listen with the mind but listen with the spirit. The function of the ear is limited to hearing; the function of the mind is limited to forming images and ideas. As to the spirit, it is an emptiness and a formlessness responsive to all things. Tao abides in emptiness; and emptiness is the fast of the mind."[12]

The act of Quranic recitation is a discipline of the mind in addition to being a form of worship in Islam. Its revelatory quality focuses the mind on the supernatural realities, and its narrative thrust and poetic ambiance actually raise the level of the mind to a higher plane of consciousness. It addition, on the sheer physical plane of experience, such recitation actually sends vibratory blessing through the entire body down to every living cell with its sacred tonality and spiritual rhythms, this being a spiritual energy force that channels itself through the physical forms of letters and words across the entire field of the human body with its blessed quality of rhythm and vibration. Needless to say, the effect of reading the revelatory Word of God permeates the mind, heart and soul of the reciter with its sublime wisdom and beatitude to the extent that the very experience of life beyond the outer shell of the body is altered with the utterance of every letter, syllable and word. Tasting, seeing, experiencing, and virtually living through the senses all demonstrate

---

12. John H. Wu, *The Golden Age of Zen* (Bloomington, IN: World Wisdom Books, 2003), p. 31.

that there is something common between our sense-experience in which we witness the existential, literal world and the enlightenment-experience in which we absorb the essence of the world as a reflection of a higher experience; the one takes place in our innermost being, the other on the fringe of our consciousness. The empirical supports the spiritual as the spokes of a wheel support the center; while the spiritual realities substantiate the empirical world of forms in the same way that fragments of transmuted light transform themselves to become the unity of a wondrous rainbow.

୭

The five senses of seeing, hearing, smelling, tasting and touching are windows of perception for outer and inner worlds, creating an ever-changing theatre of optical, auditory, gustatory, olfactory and tactile sensations and wonders that both substantiate the world and stimulate the imagination toward the world of inner experience where they ultimately find their final abode on the *tabula rasa* of the soul. Out of the sights and sounds, smells and tastes we experience the world and thus construct our souls. These windows are perennially thrown open, uncurtained and wide, in all weathers. Vision is perhaps the most expansive of the senses and has the broadest range. The human eye can roam the peaks and valleys of mountains or traverse the celestial concourse of the stars at a single glance; yet the chasm that exists between the sight of the Milky Way and its symbolic significance as a sign of a higher reality is vast and deep. Rainbows and mirages manifest under certain conditions and display themselves fleetingly for us to wonder at and behold; but their permanent image resides as an archetypal symbol and premonition of something mysterious that lies beyond the physical retinue of the eye. Both of these rarefied natural wonders inspire reverence and awe because they seem to be real, as they dissipate into the illusion that they truly are. What we take into ourselves from the natural world we use as the building blocks of a personality and a human entity that is both mysterious and unique, like no other, so that I can say to myself: this is me at any given moment, and know that there is a self identified with my existence that no one else can fully know or approximate because no one of us has sensed and taken in the world in the same manner as any other individual.

There is a boundary between myself and the world that is porous and full of holes because of the miracle of the senses and their ability to serve as windows between outer and inner worlds. As such, the soul can flow freely in and out between these two worlds, from the self out into the world of people and nature, and then back in again to the inner sanctum where experience becomes a part of the fragile texture that makes up the unique "spider web" of an individual life. The outer senses present to us some physical object that through the rarefied wonders of the senses reveals their unique, inner quality, so that the mind can separate what is sensory and material in the object from that part of the object that comes from the creative Hand and Spirit of God. When we see things, we need to stop dwelling on their "suchness" and move beyond their purely physical aspect, attempting to penetrate into their divine content, to their unseen and hidden essence. In this way, the five senses can lead toward the knowledge of God and His artifacts in this world, invoking feelings of spiritual contemplation and inciting praise of the Lord. The structure and essence of every created thing has the potential to become a book of theophany in which the Architect and Artist Himself becomes revealed as the designer and maker of all things, either manifesting His art visibly or revealing His invisible perfections through the visible, auditory, olfactory, tactile and gustatory experiences within this world. Solomon said: "By the greatness and beauty of the creatures, the Maker of them is proportionately seen." (Wisdom of Solomon 13:5)

The Quran repeatedly exhorts the true believe to pay attention to the input of the senses or asks the rhetorical question why individual entities do not take note of the implicit message of the senses, a question whose asking inspires the aspiring soul to seek its answer in the wisdom the five senses have to offer. In addition, those who have lost track of the experience of a true reality are identified as those who deny the idea of the Transcendent and the possibilities of the Spirit in principle, if such an oxymoron can be sustained without appearing truly ludicrous. They are the ones who have "lost the power to hear and they do not see" (11:20). They are said to be "blind and deaf" in comparison with those "who can see and hear well (11:24). Are they equal when they are compared? "Why then don't you take heed?" (11:24) It is interesting to note that the Quran often relies on references to seeing, hearing and the other five senses, in emphasizing the importance of recognizing the signs that abound everywhere, inspiring humanity to recognize the true reality and turn toward the God who created them. Allah himself is identified as the Ever-Watching (al-Muhaymin), the All-Seeing (al-Baseer)[13] and the All-Hearing (al-Sameer).[14]

The senses provide opportunities to drag us further into the world of the senses, casting an unrelenting grip around our daily pursuits. The Imitation of Christ warns: "The cravings of the senses drag us hither and thither, but when the hour is spent, what do you bring back with you? Remorse of conscience and dissipation of the spirit. You go out in joy and in sadness you return, and the pleasures of the evening sadden the morning."[15] Bukhari relates the traditional saying of the Prophet: "Beware! In every man's destiny there are tests of adultery. There is no running away from it. It will catch up with you." And what is precisely this adultery the Prophet Mohammed is referring to, none other than the adultery of the senses, attaining superficial satisfaction at a deep price to one's true nature. The adultery of the eyes is to look at things that lead us down a pathway toward sin. The adultery of the ears is to listen to words that will corrupt the mind and heart. The adultery of the tongue is to speak words that are untrue and have an aura about them of shadow and darkness. The Prophet warned against the shamelessness that speaks of arrogance and weakness of spirit and that represents a corruption of the use of the senses. To have a true sense of shame in the face of the Divinity, "you must guard the head on your shoulders, and the mind and thoughts in it. You must guard its seven openings: your eyes, your ears, your nostrils, and your mouth. You must guard your body and what it contains: your heart,

---

13. "Allah knows the fraud of the eyes, and all that the breasts conceal." (40:19)
14. "It is the same (to Him) whether any of you conceals his speech or declares it openly, whether he be hidden by night or goes forth freely by day." (13:10)
15. Book 1, c. xviii.

your stomach, and what is between your legs. You must guard what your hands hold and where your feet go. And remember death: that all but your soul will return to earth. Thus those who choose the eternal life in Heaven must keep under control their attachments to the attractions of this world and have shame in front of their Lord."

No one can hope to forgo the attractions of this world that appeal so forcefully to the forces of the outer senses unless he or she curbs the indulgence of the pleasure of the senses and comes to appreciate the heightened quality of the empty plains and cloudless skies that are the true ambiance of the inner senses. Each of the senses in their own unique way have the capacity to lead the soul in one of two directions, to raise us up or cast us down, by introducing to the wandering mind the lusts and tendencies that can lead to passionate attachments associated with the illusions of this world. According to the traditional perspective, the five senses place humanity in the utmost danger by their power of enslavement to the attractions of the natural rather than the supernatural world. When a physical sensation is presented to the outer senses, whether it be to see or hear, smell, taste or touch, the aspiring soul needs to separate what is sensory and material in the object that has the power to make it a reality unto itself, from that part of its essential substance that comes from the creative spirit of God. St. Paul has written in the gospels: "The invisible things of Him are clearly seen from the creation of the world, being understood by the things that are made, even His eternal power and Godhead".[16]

A true cause for joy is not the insatiable satisfaction that a physical object may contain, but rather the knowledge of God that gives the natural order of the created universe its essential quality, beauty and the wisdom of its physical form as an artifact of a higher perfection. In so doing, the outer, external aspect of the senses and their multiple attractions are neutralized, allowing the inner content of the senses, including the beauty, wisdom and perfection of natural objects to become impressed upon the mind with their inner content, leaving the soul with feelings of contentment and peace that what we see, hear, smell, taste and touch are manifestations of a

16. Romans 1:20.

Supreme Being. The level of the human mind is raised to the level of the Divine Mind to the extent that while living in the natural world, you will be able to share in the knowledge and experience belonging to a higher order of experience beyond this world. The invisible becomes visible and the inaudible becomes audible. To quote a well known Islamic tradition: "My servants continue to draw near unto Me with supererogatory works so that I shall love them. When I love them, I am the ears with which they hear, the eyes with which they see, the hands with which they strike, and the feet with which they walk." Muslims have the opportunity of presenting God's eyes and ears to the world; in return they witness the world through the eyes and ears of the Divinity.

If God whispers to us through the voice of the wind or the gurgle of a brook, do we hear the sound of the wind and the chatter of the brook or do we hear the inspirations of the Divinity making Himself known to humanity. If the image of dew on grass or the sparkle of a lake shimmering with sunlight do not haunt us with their beauty and hint of intimacy with a higher order of experience, then where can the impulses of the senses find their final abode as they flit like butterflies through the experiences of this world? When the mind is discerning and the heart is receptive to the eternal wind that passes through the temporal order as the breath of life, the soul takes wing and soars above the temporal order with detachment and grace, witnessing the world with the eternal seeing and listening and tasting that become the revelations of the other side of reality. When the Divinity sees and speaks and listens through humanity, the mystery of life is momentarily resolved and the secret is exposed to reveal an infinite joy at the heart of the life experience that justifies the effort to experience the wisdom of the senses in their natural light.

As a source of pleasure and satisfaction, we will never fully enjoy the world until we come to appreciate the resonance that each of the five senses enjoys as organs that relate directly to the inner dimensions of humanity, namely the soul and spirit of a person, awakening the inner capacity of the senses to a higher experience of reality. The senses are a venue for sacred happenings: The tranquility of an early morning fog creeping through the valley, the serene image of a snow-capped mountain peak reaching beyond the clouds; the beauty of a sacred song sung by a human voice; the taste of honey as the nectar of the angels; the smell of musk that calls to memory the divine invocation of the sacred name.[17] The senses can be raised to a higher order of magnitude and we become the grand inquisitor of all that we investigate. The senses spill their secrets into our lives as a mode of reflection and inspiration of a higher order, listening, seeing, touching, and tasting as infants do, as if for the first time, as in some primordial experience of experimentation and investigation in coming to experience the world as if it were a reflection of a higher order of experience from which we have just fallen down.

An amazing characteristic of childhood is indeed its sweet and uncomplicated naiveté that reaches out and instinctively remembers the divine source from which it has sprung. There is a wild and virgin quality to the infant soul that seems to be a direct reflection of the timeless, as if it had fallen through a crack in the fabric of eternity only to find itself encased within a body of an undeveloped baby. This is before the child can learn to consciously separate him or herself from God and attach themselves to the world. People commonly refer to childhood as the time of innocence, a time still close enough to the remembrance of the paradise lost. The innocent young soul has yet to abandon its newly lost connections with eternity, and the ambiance of the paradise and the desire to partake of its plenitude and benevolence is still instinctive and fresh. The young child is spontaneous, carefree and truthful, spontaneous in that young children live completely in the moment, carefree in that they are not burdened by the excess baggage that experience has given us, and truthful in that they show in their face the true reflection of their inner condition and not some false front with which to greet the world. A child's face is not yet molded by experience; it is a face that still lies outside of time.

---

17. Muslims place special significance in the power of scent in the remembrance (*dhikr*) of God. For this reason, sacred scents such as oud and musk, not to mention a wide variety of natural incense, are used to accompany the prayer ritual in Islam.

Children seem to live as if they belong no matter where they are and have no need to be anywhere else. They look out unconcernedly at the world around them as if they have claimed ownership and already taken possession of it. Of course they fuss when they are uncomfortable or cry when they are hungry, since the world they are beginning to experience is not the paradise they remember, but by and large they behave in that primitive infant condition with nobility and contentment, as if they have brought from their mother's womb a knowledge of their own unity, as if the sea itself flowed in its veins and a crown of stars rested fittingly on its head, as if the mystery of God's creative hand was still near at hand and the infant is still one with the Spirit of God. In the detached gaze of an infant child, the wisdom of the world is wiped clean. Watching a child at rest and free of care makes a person realize that it is not what we see, but the way we see a thing that marks the difference between a pure, virgin mentality and the corrupted, over-worldly veneer that envelopes the adult mind, trapped within a labyrinth of our own human weaknesses and weighted down by the experience of the world. In fact, what does the child see but the same world we do; but in a manner infinitely different, in which everything is at first new and strange, rare and delightful, and inexpressibly beautiful.

The infant child is a little stranger unto him or herself, but their entrance into the world is compensated by the world itself saluting them and surrounding them with innumerable joys. They know nothing of sin and regret, and they do not complain about the weather. They do not dream of poverty, contention or vice and live out of a knowledge that is instinctive and raw. Everything seems at rest, free of sorrow and having an immortal quality. They know nothing of terminal sickness or death, rents or other tributes to the hardships and turmoil of this world. All things abide eternally as if they are in their proper place. Everything is manifest in the clear light of day and behind ever created thing something infinite and eternal lies in waiting. Time for them is still a part of eternity, the universe itself is an Eden, and the world that infants experience make them heir to the mysteries which the books of the learned never unfold. They seem true to the real import of the senses in which the world is to be experience as a natural manifestation of a supernatural prototype. They have no need for words and live in the moment as if it were still part of the eternity from which they have sprung.

෴

The natural senses cannot contain the world; much less identify its reality, any more than they can possess God. As windows to and from the soul, the senses are undoubtedly in search of something, we need to identify what it is exactly that they want. "No invisible reality appears to it in a visible form. We walk by faith, not by sight."[18] St. Augustine suggests that "No one seeing God lives this mortal life in which the bodily senses have their play: and unless in some way he departs this life, whether by going altogether out of his body or by withdrawing from his carnal senses, he is not caught up into that vision."[19] The Quran refers to two definitive sides of reality. The *'alam ash-shahādah* refers to the "world of the observable" or the perceptive world pertaining to the natural, created order that we witness every day of our lives. However, certain aspects of a multi-faceted reality are beyond the reach of the outer senses of humanity. The *'alam al-ghaib* represents the "world of the mysterious" or the unseen world pertaining to the supernatural, other-worldly dimension that we experience every day of our lives, but that we don't directly witness. What the human faculty of intuition knows as a matter of spiritual instinct, the five senses are desperately in search of without finding on their own terms, namely direct knowledge, awakening to a higher reality, and transcendence. In differentiating between these two worlds, we come to realize that an unveiling is possible depending on the attitude and spirit of the individual in which one or another aspect of the "world of the unseen" may be revealed, if not to the outer senses directly, then to their inner mode of perception that permits, in addition to a direct experience of sound or scent or taste, entry to the inner side of the senses to an experience of that which is not immediately available to

18. St. Paul, 2 Corinthians 5:7).
19. *Not of this World: A Treasury of Christian Mysticism*, ed. by James S. Cutsinger (Bloomington, IN: World Wisdom Books, 2003), p. 88.

the outer senses, thus creating a heightened awareness that leads to the raising of consciousness.

The power of the senses are not confined to servicing the needs of the body only, any more than the needs of the body can determine the true nature of the cosmos through the instruments of the senses. We may split the atom in search of the building blocks of life, or search the heavens for the true moment of initial singularity; but what ultimate consequence does such a knowledge and world-view have but a listing of facts and mathematical laws that do not allow an interpretive explanation or significance beyond the realm of physical matter. Such facts certainly will never be able to define with objectivity the true nature of a reality that transcends the physical plane of existence. According to the renown imam Ghazali, the experience of *tawhīd*, which is the foundational principle of unity upon which the entire Religion of Islam is constructed, does not have to achieve the supreme act of mystical annihilation in order to comprehend its significance in principle; rather a person may experience a taste, through the unveiling of the inner senses, of supreme unity as if by the touch of some magic wand, to reveal the other side of a reality that is eternally present, but unavailable to the direct perception of the senses. The inner reality of the senses is thus unfolded to the receptive Muslim, who recites the witnessing of the sacred formula of Islam in which he or she surrenders to God (*la ilaha illa'Llah*) and then activates that surrender in practice and praise of the Divinity (*Mohammed rasul Allah*) through the path and spiritual disciplines of Islam.

We have only to imagine for a moment a life without the support of one of the senses to uncover once and for all their true value and meaning. Imagine life without the power of sight, inhabiting a living darkness amounting to an eternal night without moon or stars. Imagine a world without the power of sound that identifies the vibratory rhythm of every physical object, from the cry of the peacock to the howling of the wind through the pines. Imagine the enduring silence that would reign within our minds and hearts if the floodgates of the senses were suddenly closed and we were bereft of their implicit blessing. Suppose that the open door of the senses were suddenly closed—closed to the vision of the natural wonders of mountains, valleys and streams, cut off from the sound of song and the voices of every created object, closed to the aspirations and dreams that become a reality through the physical universe. Then it would be a silence indeed that could fill the expanse of a thousand years and span multiple universes, a silence so private and enduring it would take a forest full of trees to absorb its echoes, a silence that could only be broken by the sigh of the Great Sphinx at the resolution of its mystery. In such a world, we would be listening with full expectation, awaiting the sights, sounds and smells that truly verify the reality of our experience, not just their literal experience, but to fill our souls with the wisdom contained in the messages they convey. We would open our eyes and lift up our ears to the natural revelations of the Divinity and proclaim as in the Psalms: "We did not make ourselves, but He who endureth forever made us."[20]

As arbiters of objectivity in search of a true reality that we can believe in with confidence, the senses tell us everything we need to know about the material and natural worlds and nothing we need to know about the supernatural order of experience unless we turn their messages inward to the extent that the visible and sensible leads to an appreciation of the invisible and otherworldly, the visible sense world becomes the material reflection of an invisible supra-sensory world, conscious that what is visible is merely an image of what is invisible and that what is invisible is the archetype of what is visible. The visible, sensible, and material world is not the final destination in our search for a true reality, but rather a sign and symbol, a teacher if you will, of an invisible dimension that is the eternal dwelling-place of the Absolute and the Transcendent.

> *See, where thou nothing seest;*
> *Go, where thou canst not go;*
> *Hear, where there is no sound;*
> *Then where God speaks art thou.*[21]

---

20. Psalms, 100:3–5.

21. Angelus Silesius, *The Cherubinic Wanderer*, written under the pen name of "The Silesian Angel", quoted in *Not of this World*, ed. James S. Cutsinger (Bloomington, IN: World Wisdom Books, 2003), p.259.

On that note, I will now keep silent and bring this exposé to a close. There must be a natural limit to the extent that one can speculate and reflect upon a topic that requires direct experience in order to be fully known and internalized. Sometimes it is enough to plant a seed; the full grown tree will eventually develop of its own accord and will speak of God in its own way. If you still have a desire to read more about the wisdom secretly embedded within the five human senses, then be yourself your own book and read carefully every page. In coming to see that which is not there and to hear the inaudible that lends rhythm to the spheres and taste the incredible nectar that savors of some mysterious and unexpected truth, you will come to see true visions when nothing is there, hear resonant echoes where there is no sound, and go where you cannot go, until that moment when eternity touches time and God speaks through multiple revelations. The true dimension of your five senses will be there for you, when the voice of the Divinity breaks the enduring silence with the perennial wisdom of the ages, that when internalized will bring true happiness to the human spirit.

Let us turn our own pages and become our own book until that moment when we become once again our true selves in view of our true destiny. Let us live in reflection of that first, primordial Man, who opened the narrative of humanity to reveal the blank pages of a book that will forever record the hopes and aspirations of humanity transformed. Let us turn the experience of our lives into a process of sacred alchemy, turning uncut stones into shimmering diamonds, by recognizing through the wisdom of their senses the ineffable Spirit of God in every created thing.

2

THE VISIONARY
POWER OF SIGHT

Vision comprehends Him not,
but He comprehends (all) vision.
He is the Subtle, the Aware.
(Quran 6:103)

Throughout recorded history, vision has always distinguished itself among the five senses as the instrument of verification *par excellence*, as well as the oracular miracle that brings the wonders of the world to the inner screen of the mind. We hear a whisper of the wind, the flutter of butterfly wings, or the noisy grinding of the cicadas on a hot summer day and marvel at the variety of voices that fill the natural world with their inspired sounds. We smell burning autumn leaves or the pungent fragrance of frankincense and myrrh and are transported into the inner world of our imaginings. We taste the grapes of the vine and we feel the caress of velvet and silk. We cannot do without any one of the five senses of course without feeling a sense of great loss, whether it be the benediction of scent, the rhythms of sound or the infinitely varied flavors of taste in which the experience of the world becomes a practical reality that thrills the body as much as it overpowers the mind by inducing temptation and desire. But vision conquers all as the mighty and majestic recorder of all earthly beauties, imprinting as it does the true image of every physical form from the splendor of a bushy tree on the savannah to the exquisite cumulus clouds against a shocking blue sky. Yet, for all the cornucopia of sights that assault the mind with their visionary beauty, the act of seeing cannot comprehend the one thing needful because, as the Quran aptly reminds us: "Vision comprehends Him not, but He comprehends all vision." He is the All-Seeing and nothing escapes His all-encompassing Face (*wajh*).[1]

As much as we would like to see God, as much as we would like to reduce the unseen to a science of shape and form, as much as we would like to reduce the ineffable mystery to the primordial point hovering like the point at the end of a question mark, this will never happen, at least within the realm of reality as we experience it in this world. To see the invisible with physical eyes would neutralize the sense of the ineffable and render the visionary quest that serves as the indelible mark of our existence as void. The inner eye will not see God, angels or spirits of the non-tangible world, any more than God, one of whose names is the All-Seeing (*al-basir*), sees the world with a physical eye. Rather, because the prototype human is modelled in the image of God by reflecting His qualities and attributes, humans can fine-tune their inner senses through prayer and other spiritual disciplines, so that the human faculties can become modes of perception that lead to the inner world of higher level, spiritual experience.

The grand elements of the natural world such as mountains and oceans, rivers and forests, form a kind of phantasmagoric pictogram flashing images whose meaning gives substance to our impressions and defines the true nature of the physical world. As such, these sacred symbols constitute pieces of a grand mosaic making up the pictures of a universal exhibition, shining before our eyes in all their pristine purity as a revelatory source of knowledge about our true origins and ultimate end. I hear the sound vibrations of every living thing from the resonance of the bell to the echo of a distant flute. The world of sensation and feeling opens to me through the sense of touch to the extent that we are loved and can give love in return. When I smell a flower or freshly cut grass, the living presence of every created thing greets me with the air of its true nature and what I taste becomes the gustatory experience of the edible world. Every act of the senses is a search for the light at the center of all things from the twinkling of that distant star to the indeterminate electrons

---

1. "Wherever you turn, there is the Face of God." (2:115)

shining on a phosphorous plate, as if every created object in the natural world were a votive candle and every action induced by the senses an aspiration and prayer.

We have the sense of sight, and in particular the miracle of the human eye, to thank for the sublime vision of these natural wonders whose symbolic meaning transports us beyond the horizon of this, our beloved physical world. According to modern science, the eyes that humans enjoy find their origin in a proto-eye that evolved some 540 million years ago. The earliest eyes, called eyespots, were simple patches of photo-receptor cells, physically similar to the receptor patches that we have to facilitate the sensations of taste and smell. These eyespots could only sense ambient brightness: they could distinguish light and dark, but not the direction of the light source. In ancient seas, life forms developed faint patches of skin that were sensitive to light. Eventually, eyes evolved that could judge motion, then form, and finally a complete and dazzling array of details and colors.

The physiology of the human eye is a miracle in its own right to witness and behold. The pupil of the eye acts as a shutter to process light. The iris[2] of the eye, which is really a muscle, changes the size of a small hole, the pupil,[3] through which the light enters the eyeball. The eye's lens gathers the light and focuses it onto a thin sheet lining the rear wall of the eyeball, called the retina, to form an image. The sophisticated mechanics that permits the eye to function matches the artistry that lies embedded within the fine intricacies of the other two senses of the nose and ear. Any defect in the precision of the workings of these senses results in the loss in vision, smell or hearing. The biochemistry of vision is a staggeringly complicated process indeed and I will leave its explanation to those who are more familiar with its intricate workings. For our purposes here, it is enough to point out that, like the other senses we are exploring in this work, there is an intricate and carefully tailored outer

---

2. The iris protects against sudden surges of light and gives our eyes their color. It is named after the Greek word for rainbow.

3. From the Latin *pupilla*, "a little doll." The Hebrew expression for pupil is similar: *eshon ayin*, which means "little man of the eye."

component to the sense of sight, as well as a subtle if not more reso-
lute inner aspect to the sense of vision—tantamount to opening the
"black box of vision" to the light of a deeper and more profound
world—that has the power to see that which is invisible and hidden
from direct view, in the same way that the sense of hearing finds significance and meaning in that which is inaudible.

There is a finitude to the eye that belies its miraculous powers.
When I was younger, I had excellent vision and could literally read
in the dark as it were. But as I got older and entered into the decade
of my 40s, impending age began to show its grim face over the horizon of my life in the form of loss of vision, although hopefully it
also corresponded with a more enlightened and clearer inner vision
of which we write. I have the habit of reading when I first get up and
permit myself the torture of rising early before the sun in order to
ensure enough reading time before beginning a busy day. It was
during these extended reading sessions in the early morning that
my sight began to fail me. At first I wore reading glasses, but as the
years went by and well into my late 40s, I was already wearing my
eye glasses full time.

I had been living in Malaysia for a number of years when one day
I asked my Malay friend, who was well into his 50s, why he didn't
need glasses. In my travels, I had come across many older people
living in such places as the Middle and Far East who saw the world
through blurred vision rather than succumb to the indignity of
wearing glasses, and I thought my friend was one of them. Secretly,
I was fully expecting him to say that he couldn't see very well, but
just hadn't gotten around to getting himself a pair of glasses. As in
many other things, he surprised me with his explanation. "It wasn't
but a d-d-d-decade ag-g-ggo," he told me with his endearing stutter,
a stutter I might add that punctuated an otherwise impeccable Brit-
ish accent together with unexpected English fluency, "when I knew
for sure that I n-n-needed g-g-glasses." I will not try to recapture his
sweet and lovable style of narrative, or the gruff stuttering voice that
he delivered it; suffice it to say that he was able to glean a number of
insights from his traditional Malay culture into potential cures for a
number of ailments, one of them being poor vision. "I was t-t-t-told
to sit for an hour in the j-j-j-jungle close to the green f-f-f-foliage

for a number of d-d-d-days staring at the greenness of the l-l-l-leaves. By the end of the week, I was c-c-c-cured." He still had his stutter, and I secretly believed that it was so much apart of his unique personality that attempting to cure him of it would have robbed him of some vital aspect of his personality, and so he chose not to bother himself about it. But his vision was another thing, and this he has restored to its usual familiar clarity. Perhaps there is a message embedded with this anecdotal aside about priorities that could be useful to us all.

$$\backsim$$

For the sense of hearing, we raise the relevant question: Are we listening? For the sense of smell, we marvel at the infinite variety of odors that actually betray the inner nature of a thing. For taste, we have only to pick up a slice of pizza or dig into a juicy steak to savor the gustatory experience of food and drink. To taste, touch, smell, or hear an object, you must be relatively close to it. Vision, on the other hand, takes us by the hand and leads us headlong across oceans and mountain peaks. The blink of an eye can capture the universe in the night sky and as for the light of distant stars, they are nothing short of the graveyard of shimmering suns that happened millions of light years ago, all on offer in the gallery of stars and galaxies to our simple, unpretentious gaze. We listen to the buzzing of bees and smell the scent of jasmine in the air, but with the eyes we behold and take in the surrounding world at a glance. Even closing the eyes presents a rich array of heightened experience insofar as the sudden absence of the outer world and the plate of darkness on offer to our inner vision opens onto a world of imagination and higher intuition.

Seeing as we understand it does not happen strictly speaking in the eye but rather in the brain, and by way of extension in the mind's eye. We need only to think of the seeing that takes place in our dreams to begin to understand what it means to see with the mind's eye. Plato had an amazingly accurate perception reflective of a universal truth when he wrote several millennia ago: "It is not the eye that sees, it is the I that sees." In order to open my mind to the

"I" consciousness implicit in Plato's comment, I needed to first close my physical eyes and turn them inward to the inner "I" that represents a consciousness of self, a consciousness most notably that sets humankind apart from the rest of the creation. We must look far down into the depths of the inward self in order to ask: 'How could I make the connection and bridge the eye of the contemporary "ego" with the "I" of the eternal self that exists within me? How could I cross the chasm that exists between the "passionate and egoistic" soul (al-nafs al-ammarah) and the "soul which blames" (al nafs al-lawwamah), or the discriminating soul that the Quran so clearly identifies? How could I transform myself into a conscious being in search, not of myself and my own personal truth, but rather a conscious self in search of truth's truth? How could I become one again with the river of life that flows within me and that makes itself known as a conscious witness of all that we experience?

The Islamic traditions have an amazingly insightful saying that encaptures the mystery of faith as a source of illumination and the power of inner sight without the benefit of the eyes. "Worship Allah as if you saw Him, for even if you do not see Him, nevertheless He sees you." In the Christian tradition, Meister Eckhart echoes the same sentiment by seizing upon and capturing the essence of true vision. "The eye by which I see God is the same as the eye by which God sees me. My eye and God's eye are one and the same." Faith requires a leap of mind through the conditional "as if" in order to experience the world with the inner eye and thus to understand that which cannot be seen with the external eyes. Human beings will not see God with their eyes any more than God sees the human being with a physical "eye". To worship Allah as if we actually saw Him obliges us to dedicate ourselves to the task of imagining what is not there and then living in its presence; while in compensation, everything in the manifested universe promises to bear witness to the suggestion that something invisible is making its presence felt within us as the only enduring reality worth striving for.

These two simple words represent the supreme existential condition for the human being here on earth, a conditional that is firmly embedded within the two simple words "as if". By living one's life as if Allah actually exists, Muslims profess belief in a higher or spiritual knowledge that they cannot actually see with their own eyes, and a willingness to act upon that knowledge with a consciousness that has the power to change the course of life, much like embedded rock whose firmness can change the course of a river. That is why faithful Muslims follow the advice of their Prophet and "worship Allah as if [they] actually saw Him", because striving to worship God with the inner eye will reveal the inner spiritual dimension of the entire created universe that we witness and observe everyday as a self-evident truth.

∿

When we see a physical object or the animals within nature such as the lion or the dove, when we observe the sun, moon and stars or contemplate the great mountains, deserts and oceans; when we gaze upon a sunrise, a waterfall in the forest, or a mirage in the desert, what is it that we actually see? Is it merely the physical form that modern science has painstakingly scrutinized, identified and set in place within the natural order, or does that physical form radiate an essence and a meaning beyond the physical properties of the form? Awhadi Kirmani summarized in a four line stanza the traditional point of view regarding the world of forms that our sight partakes in.

> *I gaze upon form (surat) with the physical eye because*
> *There is in form the trace of the Spirit (ma'na).*
> *This is the world of form and we live in forms:*
> *The spirit cannot be seen save by means of form.*

Traditional symbols in the form and elements of the natural order, such as the sun, the mountains, and the horizon are found in varying degrees of importance in the symbolic language of all the revelations of the world and therefore have universal application. What we witness in nature with our eyes, just as what we hear in nature with our ears, has an importance that extends far beyond the physical form of what we see and hear, making possible the transition that needs to take place between sensible knowledge and spiritual experience. What we see has the power to speak with us; just as what we hear has the power to transport us through images and dreams beyond the rhythm of the sound. The symbolic image impresses knowledge upon us; a sound once uttered and heard has the function and power of a call, summoning us out of ourselves. A smell evokes presence and purpose, lifting us off our feet to float through the air like tendrils of smoke, to experience the very essence of a thing by virtue of its odor.

> And in the earth are signs for those whose faith is sure.
> And in yourselves. Can you then not see?
> And in the heavens is your sustenance
> and that which you are promised.
> By the Lord of Heaven and Earth,
> this is the Truth (51:20–23).

The image of the universe is a vision of the universe created in the sight of the Supreme Being, whose "Vision comprehends all vision". It is a universe defined by an infinite variety of traditional signs and symbols that confront the mind and the imagination of humanity with their revelatory knowledge of other worlds, their premonition of higher realities and their numinous message of the one supreme Reality. They exist within this world as created forms that remember God through their very existence. Through their presence, they express something of the transparent reality that exists within and beyond every external form. In fact, according to the traditionalist perspective, the entire created universe is a form of revelation and a sign of the Divinity. "Thus, we live in a fabric of theophanies of which we are a part; to exist is to be a symbol; wisdom is to perceive the symbolism of things."[4] The knowledge and grace that make up this fabric of theophanies refer to the Divinity; existence refers to everything created in the universe; wisdom refers to humanity in the form of a knowledge they are able to assimilate into their beings.

The science of symbols is virtually a traditional science of sacred realities, a science of inner qualities and sacred attributes, that extends far beyond the purely physical form of the symbols within the world of nature. Symbols do not have as their function and purpose the exposition of a graphic picture or a pretty sound. A chain

4. Frithjof Schuon, *Roots of the Human Condition* (Bloomington, IN: World Wisdom Books, 1991), p. 57.

of mountains or a brilliant sunset is not just beautiful in and of itself. A symbol signifies the articulation of a truth and the identification of a reality that is supra-natural and beyond the formal plane of earthly manifestation, the suggestion of an inner world embedded within its outer form. The clarity and vividness of such symbols as the Hand of God, the Edenic Tree, and the Divine Light contain an arresting power that seizes human imagination with its suggestive mystery of a higher reality, as well as the mystery of creation, of knowledge, and of enlightenment. Sweeping deserts, vast oceans and the vault of heaven overwhelm the human mind not only with their magnitude, as in the numerical projections of modern science, but also with their power to produce meaning and induce reflection. They were never intended to be mere form, as they are understood in today's world of science. Rather, they exist as outward manifestations of the power and omnipotence of the Divinity so that humans could gain access to the inner meaning behind the phenomena of nature, thus neutralizing the tyranny of the literal form with its sacred and beatitudinal inner reality.

Symbols are a form of revelation and thus a primary source of knowledge for humanity. They exemplify in sheer form supra-rational possibilities that form the basis of understanding of the true nature of reality. They reflect multiple layers of reality for traditional man and relate directly to our spiritual intuition and instincts. Moreover, they are the means for the communication of a truth that would otherwise be inexpressible, a truth whose fundamental character would defy analysis because its reality is a mystery that lies beyond the range of ordinary language and beyond the power of ordinary discursive thought. Every pictorial image in the creation has a qualitative aspect embedded with the graphic and often sonorous form.[5]

In other words, symbols convey a broad range of meaning extend-

---

5. Symbols are not only visual images. They can be sounds (a mantra is a sound symbol), language (a word is an auditory symbol written down as a graphic image), a gesture, rites and rituals, sacred art, and the crafts. In other words, they can be visual, as in nature, sacred art and language; auditory as in sound, words, and music; olfactory, as in a variety of scents, including perfume and incense.

ing far beyond their literal form. They are as old as the tree, as sacred as fire, as powerful as water and as mysterious as the veil. They are as enduring as marble, as beautiful as the rose, as peaceful as the dove, and as timely as the Final Hour and the Last Day. They lead beyond the surface of things and give entrance to the realms of an unseen reality. As a vehicle of knowledge, symbols are a veil, a mirror and a key. They are the protective veils of the knowledge of God, the mirrored reflection of the ideas and archetypes within higher reality, and the keys to the understanding of the fundamental mystery that underlies everything in the manifested world.

Every manifested form and every created thing not only exists and has meaning; but also participates in the Transcendent Principle. That is the primary meaning of the truth in the Quranic verse which states that everything in the created universe prays and praises the Divinity in a form of worship that is ontological and universal. "Whatever is in the heavens and on the earth doth declare His praise and Glory and He is the Exalted in might, the Wise" (59:24). In other words, existence itself is prayer and praise. The gnat (and other insects), the atom and the date-palm seed (and other seeds such as grain *et. al.*) are singled out in the Quran, the atom representing the smallest yet most powerful source of energy, the seed the basic life-giving and fructifying element.

Even the lower forms of life, such as the gnat,[6] the spider,[7] and the fly[8] can serve as an example to humanity, seemingly insignificant creatures that can also convey a higher relevance and meaning. The very dust at our feet forms one of the basic elements of man's

6. "Allah does not disdain to use the similitude of things, lowest (the gnat) as well as the highest. Those who believe know that it is truth from their Lord. But those who reject faith say: 'What means Allah by this similitude?'" (2:26).

7. "The parable of those who take protectors other than Allah is that of the spider who builds itself a house; but truly, the flimsiest of houses is the spider's house" (29:41).

8. "O men! Here is a parable set forth! Listen to it! Those on whom you call, besides Allah, cannot create (even) a fly, if they all met together for the purpose. And if the fly should snatch away anything from them, they would have no power to release it from the fly. Feeble are those who petition and those whom they petition!" (22:73)

formative primordial development. "Among His signs is that He created you from dust (30:20) and unto dust, the proverbial adage
reminds us, we shall return. When we die and become dust and
bones, shall we indeed receive rewards and punishments?" (37:53)
Created from dust, man gains value by reflecting the Divine Light
that shines through him, for even a speck of dust reflects a beam of
sunlight upon the breast of its existence. Ultimately, on the Day of
Judgment, when those who denied the truth are faced with "that
which they have their hands have sent forth, they will cry out the
final humiliation: I wish I were dust (78:40). As an end in themselves, created forms are contingent, superficial, and insignificant; as
symbols of a higher reality, they are generous, eloquent and profound. All natural phenomena can be regarded from two perspec-
tives, the physical object with a practical utility and the metaphysical
symbol with an ultimate significance, while the symbolic aspect
constitutes its most fundamental and profound reality.

All of the elements of virgin nature still retain in principle the
primordial qualities of beauty, serenity and holiness that humans
seeks and can find within the sacred symbols of the world of nature
if they share in the symbolist sympathy for the messages that are
implicit within this natural environment. The silence of forests, the
majesty of distant mountains, and the brilliance of the setting sun
witness and testify to the holiness and the healing factors that are
the inherent properties within nature and point to the spiritual
presence that can calm disquieted minds and balance the disharmony of unhappy souls. The yearning to return to nature that we
witness during these times reflects the deep-seeded yearning for the
beauty, tranquillity and peace that are fundamental desires of
human nature, but that are far distant memories for modern individuals who must cope in their daily lives with the debilitating ugli-
ness of the world and the stressful complexity of life in our huge,
impersonal and virtually inhuman metropolises.

❧

Traditional symbols can be characterized primarily by their beauty
and their efficacy. Firstly, the symbol can be called beautiful by

virtue of its actually "being" what it gives expression to and represents, namely a spiritual truth and a higher reality that is reflected within the form. "A symbol is not something arbitrarily chosen by man to illustrate a higher reality; it does so precisely because it is rooted in that reality, which has projected it, like a shadow or a reflection, onto the plane of earth."[9] In other words, we say that a symbol is beautiful primarily because it is true. The beauty of an object results from the transparency of its form through which a truth is made known, and there is nothing more beautiful than a truth that is made manifest. Secondly, a symbol can be called beautiful because it has a universal character and says something of the Unity that lies at the heart of the universe and is its mirror reflection in form. "The beauty of a thing is the sign of its internal unity, its conformity with an indivisible essence, and thus with a reality that will not let itself be counted or measured."[10]

A machine,[11] for example, is not beautiful, although it is the conventional symbol *par excellence* for the modern world, full of utility and efficiency, but totally lacking in the subtlety, grace and truth traditionally associated with beauty. It may be efficient, functional, utilitarian, economical, and technologically advanced, to name its most obvious qualities; but it does not reflect a truth or identify a spiritual reality. A swan,[12] on the other hand, incarnates within its very form an aspect of dignity that is virtually archetypal. By isolating this formal aspect of perfection within an animal, it makes the animal not only beautiful, but also symbolic of a higher spiritual quality. There is an entire range of animals that actually project direct and immediate impressions of a symbolic nature. These ani-

9. Martin Lings, *the Eleventh Hour: The Spiritual Crisis of the Modern World in the Light of Tradition and Prophecy* (Cambridge, UK: QuintaEssentia, 1987), p. 36.

10. Titus Burckhardt, *Mirror of the Intellect* (Albany, NY: SUNY Press, 1987), p. 33.

11. It could be argued that a machine is a symbol, because it is a form that represents an idea concerning means and end that is realized with precision if not with grace. A traditional symbol is not an earthly form created for merely a pragmatic and utilitarian end; rather it is a formal means to a spiritual end.

12. In the Hindus tradition, the divine swan Hamsa, swimming on the primordial sea, hatches the golden egg of the world.

mals highlight for humanity one of the higher qualities or other-worldly attributes toward which we aspire, the intrinsic beauty of a symbol lying in its meaning and in its truth rather than in its form *per se.*

The lamb and the dove, in addition to the swan, are animals that project a quality of innocence and peace that borders on the other-worldly, while their white color is suggestive of celestial purity. The owl projects wisdom through its "image" and physicality, without the wherewithal for actually being wise. The bear manifests an aspect of heaviness and cunning, and it literally retreats into the earth (cave) for its winter hibernation. The squirrel, on the other hand, elfin and almost cherubic in appearance, shrewdly gathers and stores its nuts for the winter, and remembers where they are when it needs them. Who can look upon the astute activity of the squirrel and not wish to incorporate this proverbial quality into themselves? The camel suggests patience and contemplation, not to forget its ascetic aspect that is curiously reflective of the harsh environment of the desert where the camel thrives. The bee[13] is an "inspired" animal that produces honey through its "instinctive" intelligence and whose skill in house building reflects the divine wisdom. The ant,[14] a lowly creature indeed, was honored by Solomon. The ant, among other social insects, has been a source for all kinds of parables, giving lessons in industry, interdependence, altruism, frugality, humility, patience and endurance. All of these animals reflect at least one of the higher qualities towards which humans aspire and, in endeavoring to exist through the instinctive animal intelligence granted by God, they express their individual symbolic qualities to perfection and without compromise.

13. "And thy Lord taught the bee to build its cells in hills, on trees, and in habitations; then to eat of all the produce of the earth, and find with skill the spacious paths of its Lord. There issues from within their bodies a drink of varying colors wherein is a healing for me: verily in this is a sign for those who give thought." (16: 68) Most notably, the entire Sura 16 of the Quran is named *al-Nahl*, the bee.

14. "At length, when they came to a (lowly) valley of ants, one of the ants said: 'O yea ants, get into your habitations, lest Solomon and his hosts crush you (under foot) without knowing it.'" (27:18) The entire Sura 27 of the Quran is named *al-Naml*, the Ants.

In addition to the engaging symbolism of the animal kingdom, the symbols of nature are stunningly beautiful and virtually define the meaning of beauty. Anyone who has witnessed the drama of a sunset, the enchanting quality of the night sky, or the artistry of a snow crystal knows what the beauty of nature can be and is. Yet, how is it possible to further articulate this beauty in words when the symbols themselves serve this purpose so magnificently? The qualities of nature's beauty and therefore nature's truth are reflected firstly in its sense of order and harmony, which by implication conveys to humanity a feeling of certitude that behind this order lays an imperial law that is reflective of a Divinity who has created these awesome phenomena. To participate in the world of nature creates a sense of peace that leads to tranquility of mind and serenity of heart.

In addition, nature conveys the unmistakable impression of sacredness and primordiality. That is why it always produces a spiritual experience that borders on instinctive worship of the Unseen Reality by conveying the feeling that, through the open face of nature, we have has witnessed indirectly the clear Face of the Divinity. The grandeur of the primeval forest, the majesty of the open seas, the vastness of the heavens, and the sublime wonder of the night sky all induce higher levels of awareness through such spiritually emotive experience, the reason being that these symbols all reflect higher levels of reality and indeed the Divine Being Himself Who has created that reality. As such, all of nature, what we refer to endearingly as Mother Nature, transcends the normal modes of symbolic expression because Nature is actually beautiful beyond words and beyond belief.

Consider, for example, the elements and substances of nature, how they have developed and grown within certain optimal conditions that were conducive to their order and design. Is this pattern of development an accident, a chance happening, some form of necessity as many modern scientists would have us believe, or are we dealing once again with the miracle of the creation symbolized by the Hand of the Divinity. We only need to think of the great substances of nature such as diamonds, gold, silver and other natural elements, how beautiful and desirable they have always been. Think of the qualities of such precious stones as the transparent crystallinity of diamonds, the bold color of emeralds, sapphires and rubies, the perfection of pearls, and the solidity and smoothness of marble. Even the varieties of wood that characterize certain trees make statements that extend far beyond the literal constitution of the tree. We are thinking here, for example, of the majesty of the oak, the dignity (and scent) of pine, the verticality of the poplar, and the ethereality of the willow. All these objects within nature are natural and pure, without artifice or pretense. They express integrity and completeness, and they speak a message to all those who appreciate these natural images and substances, a message expressed most eloquently through the voice of silence. Precious stones in particular are known to have a unique resonance whose sympathetic vibration can have a soothing, even healing effect on a person. Ivory has traditionally been used for carving exquisite statuettes and other handicrafts because of its unusual color and pliability; while marble has provided the source material for ancient monuments and world renowned sculptures because of the implicit beauty of its configuration, its integrity of stone, and its simplicity and purity. Wood has traditionally been associated with the sense of smell or taste. Pine is remembered for its exquisitely odoriferous scent evoking the mysterious lure of the woodland forest; frankincense is the solidified sap of a tree found in Oman; Vermont maple syrup is an edible sap drawn from the inner seams of the maple tree.

Ultimately, the beauty of a traditional symbol lies in its efficacy, and its qualities are essentially threefold. The symbol is simple, it is universal, and providentially it is true.

Like all spiritual knowledge and its corresponding wisdom, the symbol is first of all simple, yet profound. For those sensitive to their intuitive message, the traditional symbol moves from the outer world of man to the interior plane of human consciousness with immediate impact. Its simple, clear image appeals first to the eye with its incarnate image and its veiled meaning. Its picturesque impression then moves quickly inward from eye to mind to heart to soul. It imprints itself on the retina before opening and expanding the mind to the substantive meaning of the symbol. Beyond eye and mind, the message of the symbol proceeds inward to the heart wherein spiritual sensibility and intuition come into play in order to transform the literal meaning of the symbol, whether it be an image, a word, a sound, a gesture, or a spiritual rite, into an irresistible and intuitive impression of the Higher Reality whose remembrance takes root and proliferates in the ground of the human soul.

Because of their fundamental simplicity and directness of projection, symbols help clarify the mystery of the world. Admittedly, we are perennially in doubt about our origins, our purpose on earth, and our ultimate end. In addition, we are forced to acknowledge the truth of an all-pervasive mystery that lies at the core of manifested existence and defies all logical explanation. The profound simplicity and directness of symbols clarifies—through an image, a gesture, a word, or a sound—an idea or an aspect of knowledge that would otherwise be inaccessible to our shallow minds. They have the power to summarize and condense within form the very essence of a meaning that may otherwise elude our intellectual grasp, particularly in this day and age when we think with our minds rather than with our hearts, unlike the people of more traditional times, for whom the heart was the virtual "seat" of the intelligence.

The symbol is not a rational definition and as such, it does not suffer the limitations that purely rational thinking exhibits. Symbols are descriptive, not argumentative. They are affirmations rather than theories and convey a graphic meaning by way of illustration through pictures, gestures, or words, and not through rational arguments and sensory proofs. Definitions and meanings that are the result of a purely rational mind organize concepts according to their logical and purely rational implications, but they do not leave an open door to an extended reality beyond the limitations of the mind. The symbol, on the other hand, while it does not lose any of its precision or directness, remains openly "vertical" and is a key to the supra-rational realities that would otherwise be beyond our conceptual and cognitive reach. The symbol is neither rational nor irrational, as some might suggest; rather it is supra-rational and vertical.

Moreover, the simplicity of the symbol embodies a profundity of meaning. Its image contains an extraordinary power to summarize within an understandable frame of reference a profound concept. It has the power to call to mind the archetypes that correspond to ideas and intellections that lie beyond the human plane. Archetypes belong to the realm of pure spirit and are reflected on the psychic plane as virtualities of deeper concepts that eventually become crystallized as actual images in the real world. They provide a graphic and distinctive explanation to the human mentality of a reality that must remain veiled from direct view. In this way, humanity generally can gain access to spiritual insights concerning the mysteries and the true nature of reality as long as individuals are open and receptive to the natural symbols that abound in the world of nature. It is as if an understanding of the value of the science of symbols and its corresponding symbolic language opens the door to an unexpected but welcome insight. If you could effectively read the message of symbols, would this give access to the totality of the truth that lay behind these earthly images? If you understood the principial knowledge behind the import of symbols, would the wisdom of the world become apparent as well? If you could know in your inner being one thing fully, could you, in a manner of speaking, know everything?

Even universal questions require individual answers; that is why the answers implicit in individual symbols convey universal meaning. Beyond their beauty, efficacy and simplicity, symbols project a quality of universality that complements their quality of profound simplicity. They are not bound to any individual religion; that is why they are referred to as traditional and not religious. When people are moved by a symbolic image, gesture, word or sound, they don't think they have something to do with religion; they think they have something to do with truth, reality, and the spirit, all of which transcend the individual forms of the religions. The picturesque and symbolic image of the mountains has always called to mind "the heights" and the proximity to Heaven. Perhaps that is why mountain climbers have always attempted to scale their peaks, often without fully knowing why. People have admired or attempted to climb mountains throughout the ages because they represent the abode of the gods. To climb a mountain was to approach the Principal and the Presence.

The image of the heavens has always presented an immediate image of the cosmic universe and its seven heavens have always conjured up the idea of the multiple layers of reality that are manifested both within and beyond the human plane. The Divine Throne prevalent within the Christian and Islamic traditions summons to mind the cosmic power, authority and dominion of the Divinity, as the renown Throne Verse (2:255) in the Quran attests: His "Throne doth extend over the heavens and the earth." The sun universally exhibits centrality and luminosity and among the various traditions, it represents the Universal Intellect, while the moon has traditionally been associated with the beauty of the beloved because of its pale, reflective light. The sacred Tree of Life is a concept that goes back to ancient times, rooted to the earth but with its branches reaching for the heavens. It features in both the Christian and Islamic traditions as the pivotal image of knowledge and life. Adam was tempted with the Tree of Eternal Life and because of his fatal choice it became for him the Tree of Knowledge between Good and Evil.

One of the greatest symbols of all time, widely recognized because of its comprehensiveness and universality is the symbol of the veil which, as *maya* in Hinduism and as *al-hijab* in Islam, plays an important role in Middle-Eastern as well as in Oriental metaphysics. Humanity is veiled from the immediate and direct perception of the spiritual realities through a formal and manifested world that is in itself a veil. This veil is increasingly opaque during this time period because the modern mentality exhibits a narrow understanding of reality as embodied within the framework of modern science, a science that refuses to recognize the transparency of the world and settles instead for the literal interpretation of the world as a reality unto itself.

The veil has been traditionally understood as being two-edged in its meaning and implications. On the one hand, the veil acts as a solid barrier to further insight in which no penetration into the true nature of reality is possible, such as we find during these times. The veil of knowledge protects itself from the uninitiated, the unwilling, and the unfaithful. On the other hand, the veil also serves as an open door, such as we find in the science of symbolism and within the symbolist spirit, and becomes transparent so that a human intuition and an appreciation for the higher realities can become possible for the human mentality that is willing to lift the veil. Thus, the veil of knowledge within the traditional framework both protects and reveals, and the veil of the world both hides and manifests the true nature of reality.[15] In Islam, one of the Holy Traditions states:

"God has seventy thousand veils of light and darkness; were He to draw their curtain, then would the splendors of His Face (*wajh*) surely consume everyone who apprehended Him with his sight." Also, the archangel Gabriel has said: "Between me and Him are seventy thousand veils of light." In the ancient Egyptian traditions, no one shall lift the veil of Isis. Isis is "all that has been, all that is and all that shall be;" and "no one hath ever lifted my veil."

Water is the Great Purifier of body and soul, the universal symbol of purity and purification. For the Hindus, the waters of life find their embodiment in the River Ganges, whose source resides in the eternal ice of the Himalayas, the mountains of the gods and the roof of the world. Whoever bathes in the Ganges is freed from all sins. Water also symbolizes the *materia prima* of the whole universe. In the Bible, the Spirit of God moved upon the face of the waters, while the Quran reconfirms this truth with the words "and His Throne was over the waters" (11:7). In addition, Quranic scripture asserts that "We have made from water every living thing" (21:30) and "He sends down water from the skies, and the channels flow, each according to its measure" (13:17). Everything in nature speaks the truth, proclaims the Divinity, and reflects the inner reality through the expression of natural forms. All the miracles that the eye perceives within the natural order begin as a mystery of creation and ends as a proof of God.

One final example may serve to highlight the broad nature and universality of the traditional symbols. We refer to the well-known symbol of the mirror that has been referred to as "the symbol of the symbol."[16] Symbolism generally provides an ambience that creates

15. "In a symbol there is concealment and yet revelation: here therefore, by silence and by speech acting together, comes a double significance.... In the symbol proper, what we can call a symbol, there is ever, more or less distinctly and directly, some embodiment and revelation of the Infinite; the Infinite is made to blend itself with the Finite, to stand visible, and as it were, attainable there. By symbols, accordingly, is man guided and commanded, made happy, made wretched." Thomas Carlyle, a Scottish essayist of the 19th century, in his *Sator Resartus*, bk. 3, chap. 3, as quoted in *The Columbia Dictionary of Quotations* (New York, NY: Columbia University Press, 1995).

16. Titus Burckhardt, *The Mirror of the Intellect* (Albany, NY: SUNY Press, 1987).

within our daily lives a symbolic link with the Transcendent and unconditional Reality of which our relative reality is but a reflection. Symbols provide a visible and graphic reflection of ideas and archetypes that cannot be fully expressed in words. St. Paul summarized it succinctly in this well known quote from the New Testament: "For now we see through a glass, darkly; but then face to face: now I know in part; but then shall I know even as also I am known." (Cor. 13:12) Within the Buddhist tradition, a teaching from *Ch'an* Buddhism concerning the implications of the mirror states: "Just as it is in the nature of a mirror to shine, so all beings at their origin possess spiritual illumination. When, however, passions obscure the mirror, it becomes covered over, as if with dust." (*Tsung-mi*). Within the Islamic perspective, according to a saying of the Prophet Mohammed, there is "for everything a means of polishing it and freeing it from rust. One thing alone polishes the heart, namely the remembrance of God (*dhikr Allah*)." The world, and humans who lives in that world, are both a veil and a mirror, veil through sheer physical form that conceals the truth from direct perception, and mirror that transcends the physical form through its symbolic projection and finds its existence in God. The universe as macrocosmic mirror is the universal body of God, just as the human being as microcosm is made in the "image" of God and as mirror reflects God's qualities and attributes.

One final attribute of the traditional symbol and its most endearing characteristic needs mentioning, in addition to its beauty and its universality. A symbol is ultimately true because it represents a truth. It brings a veiled reality of the Divine Mystery down into the world of humanity in order to make it a living reality through images, symbols, signs, and substances of the natural and visible world. The essence of their truth and their immediate reality formalizes the objective reality that they remember and reaffirm. Above all, the truth implicit in symbols has the power of transforming the modern mind, whose secular vision perceives the world in all the density of its physical projection, into a symbolist spirit whose vision perceives the world as a reflection and remembrance of the Higher Reality. By witnessing the world of forms as symbols of a higher reality and as mirrors of a higher knowledge, modern individuals can once again see eternity in time, the absolute in the relative, spirit in form, and thus transform the temporal shapes of natural phenomena into timeless symbols of reality.

~

A question that hovers in the background of our imagination or that stands on the edge of the horizon of our known world is one that strikes at the heart of who we are: How goes my world and what does it mean? We see it readily enough spread out before us with our own two eyes as an intractable zone of terrain clear to the horizon as well as the farthest reaches of the imagination. While we pretend that the vision of this physical world offers a satisfying objectivity about the true nature of reality, we are still left with the same feelings of emptiness and extreme aloneness that we experience when we see the great globe of the earth on its solitary orbit through dark outer space. It is almost as if we need to put our physical senses to sleep in order to awaken the inner eye to see that which is invisible and to elevate ourselves above the light of rational understanding in order to arrive at the enlightenment of a higher spiritual experience. No matter what we see here on earth with the physical eye, we instinctively continue to follow in the footsteps of those who have gone before us in search of that fertile valley or that glaciered mountain peak shimmering with ice, in search of a true vision about ourselves that could become a part of our external lives.

Traditional civilizations were no stranger to the possibilities of the inner, the third eye. No traditional symbol captures the mystery and the essence of the other side of reality hidden from our direct view than the symbolism of the eye. We are familiar with the everyday references to the eye of the needle and the eye of the storm. The Quran itself[17] makes reference to the fact that there will be no passing through the gates of heaven for the arrogant and those who do not appreciate the signs and symbols of nature until the camel

---

17. To those who reject Our signs and treat them with arrogance, no opening will there be of the gates of heaven, nor will they enter the garden, until the camel can pass through the eye of the needle: Such is Our reward for those in sin. (7:04)

can pass through the eye of the needle. The implication remains that those enter the paradise will be akin to having passed through the eye of a needle, in addition to having crossed the infamous bridge that crosses the chasm between heaven and hell. While the eye of the needle recalls impossibility and precision, the eye of the storm calls to me the serenity and sense of presence required to pass through the turmoil of life's vicissitudes.

Just as the physical eye opens its lid to behold the panoramic beauty of the world of nature, so also the inner eye lifts a veil in the heart to behold intuitively the imaginal world of the Invisible Realm. The symbol of the "eye of the heart"[18] is not confined to the Islamic tradition, but has a universal appeal that cuts across the broad spectrum of the various traditions. Plato mentions the "eye of the soul", St. Augustine *oculus cordis*,[19] not the mention the "third eye" that we are familiar with in the Hindu and Buddhist doctrines. The eye of the heart is actually the symbolic representation of the intellect, a faculty that is able to perceive (see) God spontaneously and without interference. It is the "eye" so to speak that will not only see the invisible world but ultimately God, the same eye no less in which God sees us. As such the eye of the heart occupies a kind of borderland between two worlds, the one external and visual and the other internal and visionary.

Within the traditional perspective, the heart lies within a borderland between two visions of a single reality. One of these visions gazes outward upon the world in order to witness there an indirect image of the reality through the symbols and signs of nature that amount to a premonition of what lies behind that image. The other vision gazes inward toward the sacred center of man's personal, inner world in order to experience directly within the heart the universal vision of the one true reality. As such, the heart has a dual role and therefore a dual meaning. As the center of the individual in

18. *'Ayn al-qalb* in Arabic and *chishm-I dil* in Persian
19. "Our whole business therefore in this life is to restore to health the eye of the heart whereby God may be seen;" (The Confessions), and in Plato: "There is an eye of the soul which . . . is more precious by far than ten thousand bodily eyes, for by it alone is truth seen." (*Republic* VII, 527E)

view of the outer world, it expresses the broad range of the human emotions based on the faith it expresses and the knowledge it chooses to believe in. As the center of the individual in view of the inward dimension, however, it expresses its true centrality as the human microcosm of the transcendent Principle. It becomes the eye that sees and the seat that discerns and bears witness to the truth of the one Reality.

We have then a case for two visions, the one external in order to view the world, the other internal in order to form the vision of a rarefied universe that intuits the knowledge of God and irradiates His presence throughout the presence of the human being. Meister Eckhart wrote in the Middle Ages many centuries ago: "The soul has two eyes—one looking inwards and the other outwards. It is the inner eye of the soul that looks into essence and takes being directly from God." More poignantly, perhaps, we need to include a comment by the American transcendentalist Ralph Waldo Emerson who wrote: "Standing on bare ground, my head bathed by the blithe air and uplifted into infinite space, all mean egotism vanishes. I become a transparent eyeball; I am nothing, I see all; the currents of the Universal Being circulate through me; I am part or parcel of God."[20] As organ of man and symbol of the Divinity, the eye passes through various modalities of expression. In man is the capacity to see; but this does not mean that there is only one level of seeing: what he sees, how he sees it and what is the result of his sight depends on his capacity to open his eyes to the shades and degrees of light and shadow depending upon the medium through which he sees. In traditional parlance, the heart is a medium of sight for the purposes of inward vision.

Traditional peoples, who understood themselves to be spiritual beings first and foremost, worshipped the Divine Being with a faith and a vigilance that implied an inward seeing with the eye of the heart, a direct and convincing vision if there ever was one. The essential knowledge of God that descended to earth through revelation was accessible to them as a matter of spiritual instinct. They

---

20. Quoted in Loren Eiseley's *The Star Thrower* (New York, NY: Harcourt, Brace and Company, 1978), p. 211.

not only enjoyed sight, but also a deep vision that allowed them to penetrate into the meaning behind the formal and manifested world of Nature. This inner eye of the heart plays a crucial role in understanding the true nature and role of the human being in the earthly sphere of existence. It is the eye of hope that ultimately offers a vision of certainty. The spiritual challenge of traditional and contemporary peoples is to reopen the eye of the heart, or to liberate their intelligence so that it can perceive once again the spiritual verities that were once "second nature" to more traditional peoples.

On the surface of life, we are never fully sure of ourselves and the questions that occasionally rise to the surface only to sink back into the dark depths of the inner self and never fully go away. Do we look out onto the world with the cold indifference of a physical eye or is there a 'transparent eye' within us whose perception and understanding makes a sacred niche of the world, in which everything is holy, reflects a knowledge of the Divinity and is a symbolic remembrance of God. Despite the enormous immensity of the phenomenal universe, with its myriad stars and galaxies strewn across a vast heaven representing incalculable distances,[21] the world of space, time and matter is not enough for humanity, not because it isn't vast or long or solid enough, but because the immensity and implications of the universe are incalculable and leave us numb and cold in terms of its significance and meaning. We cannot adhere to a faith in its exclusive reality because we are not sure what it offers us in and of itself. We sense on some instinctive level that we are not fully contained within its dimensions and that we extend somewhere else outside and beyond the physical continuum of the universe. Unless we open the inner eye of the heart, we will never perceive the symbolic meaning of the dark night with its shimmering worlds and we will never escape beyond the edge of the horizon

---

21. We don't even realize it, but to gaze upon the night sky with the twinkling light of far distant galaxies is actually like looking into a vast archeological site of the universe. What we are witnessing is actually the residue of light that has travelled billions of light years to reach our casual glance and is therefore equally as old. To truly witness the momentality of the night sky would take another few billion years.

that ultimately leads to the truth that lies within the "eye of certainty". "Indeed this is the very Truth and a certainty" (56:95).

Truth is like a crystal, many-sided, multi-angled, impenetrable and brilliant, sending rays of light from the eye of certainty into the eye of the heart. The question remains: Do we see the truth when it presents itself in the world of forms? Without the benefit of the symbolic "eye" we have written about, the unflinching certainty of the truth fluctuates widely between that which is obvious and that which is hidden. In fact, truth passes through phases of perception in human eyes that appear as obvious, universal, mysterious, enigmatic, and hidden.

Truth alone remains obvious enough to make itself accessible to the mass of humanity at all levels of the human spectrum. Truth alone is universal enough in its overall appeal to be able to penetrate the hearts of all people unconditionally, even if during these times many individuals elect not to partake of its rich possibilities through a traditional, religious faith. Truth alone contains a mystery that allows us to fulfil our role as the most pretentious creature in God's creation insofar as we ignore the essence of a truth that saves. Truth alone remains enigmatic enough to keep some people "guessing", in addition to creating the conditions of a challenge that maintains the precarious balance of certainty and doubt within the human condition. Finally, truth alone is hidden enough to remain closed off from the ignorant and protected from the evil-hearted.

Ultimately, truth is the Reality beyond human reckoning that awaits the signature of faith that sees with the inner eye that which cannot be seen with the outer eye. "Happy is the man who can open the eyes of his heart with the aid of Heaven before his earthly eyes become shut at the moment of death, and who is able to see the countenance of the Beloved while still possessing the precious gift of human life." In the end, we open our own inner eye on our own. No one can explain to another the mysterious silence that descends upon us when we kneel down to pray. We need to listen on our own in order to hear. No one can explain the vision of the invisible when we seek to understand the reality beyond the edges of our dreams. There is always something left unsaid and unseen, an echo of some high premonition and a vision of some higher reality that remains when the echo of words have disappeared and the mirage of this world has vanished. We journey through life in search of a vision that gives expression to what lies beyond the solitary realm of the mind and heart. In journeying to the end of the earth, we may ultimately find that we only needed to open our eyes to discover what we were looking for.

3

THE EVOCATIVE
POWER OF SCENT

Through the forgetfulness we seek from counterfeit delights,
Amidst our frenzies comes, more virginal and sweet,
The melancholy scent of lilacs.
(Henri de Regnier)

A careful study of the dusky archives of history both ancient and
modern reveals a human fascination with the undeniable powers
of scent. The varied aspects of its mystery, its beauty, and its refusal
to give up its dark and ethereal secrets have captured the minds
and hearts of people everywhere down through the ages. Men and
women throughout history have sought a variety of ways to fulfill
their instinctive desire to raise their spirits and smell the scents of
the paradise. In today's environment, with its secular worldview and
the propensity of people the world over to base much of their understanding of the reality of the world on the perception, if not the raw
experience, of their senses, scent has undoubtedly played a predom-
inant role in the way humans define their experience of the world.

Scent is nothing if not provocative, evocative, erotic, compelling,
alluring, pungent, disgusting, revolting, nauseating, and sickening,
creating a virtual drama of conflicting emotions that set the scene
and color our reactions to every experience from eating to intimacy.
Adjectives abound in every language that endeavor to articulate in
words the essence of a meaning that captures the quality at the heart
of a particular scent, running the gambit from the sublime to the
revolting. Just read the attempted description on the back of French
wine label to appreciate the extend people will go in their attempt to

describe the impossible. Scent projects into the air, then into the nose, and ultimately the human sensibility the aromatic essence of a thing with its summative statement "this is what I am and this is what I have to offer." There is no secret to the knowledge, and its fascinating history will verify, that the human sense of smell contains evocative powers that can raise the human sensibility on high to the very threshold of the paradise or cast the anguished mind down into the depths of the realm of revulsion and despair from which they may never fully return, all attributable to the incredible range of octave notes on the scale of olfactory sensation. From the sublime to the repulsive, we smell our way through the approbation and censure of our experiences of the world. Through smell, we can identify the true polarity of any olfactory experience in life.

There is a fleeting quality to the sense of smell that leaves us unsatisfied and longing for more, provided it emanates from the pole of pleasure; from the pole of displeasure, we flee in horror from its corrupting wake. It is as if a given scent has no true history and not recognizable future; but rather lives only in the present moment. The smell of the lilac and the distinctive odor of burning autumn leaves was the same during the time of the Roman Empire as it was on the streets of New England last fall. Only the immediate experience gives value to its name as its remembrance disappears into the void. While odors linger, they do not last and they are almost impossible to resurrect through memory even if a given scent sends memory afloat through a labyrinth of forgotten remembrances. On the contrary, their distinctive odors evoke memory and serve as a strong remembrance of that which is associated with its distinctive scent, and yet we cannot fully remember the essence of a scent until it makes itself known and we experience it again, reviving its history once again into an immediate experience we cannot deny. From an evolutionary point of view, the power of scent is one of the most ancient of the senses, the primitive sense if you will, that served as a means of identification for food, people, predators, pleasure, pain, danger. If the sense of smell is well tuned, as we expect all the senses were in more primitive times, as with wild animals not to mention proto-forms, it is an effective instrument through which the environment and the natural order communicate with us their hidden secrets.

There is an intensity to the sense of smell and the odors that invade the olfactory canals that leaves us wondering if it is possible to have too much of a good thing. All of the five senses are conduits of things whose ultimate destination we never seem to reach, so that when we do fall victim to some chance intensity of sound or smell, we can wonder if enough is already too much. We have a hint of something sweet or sour, brash or revolting; but we never fully arrive on the other side of the smell and perhaps that is a mercy in itself. The scent of jasmine is glorious, but we could only stand so much and we sense an instinctive limit; we do not want to arrive at the heart of the jasmine flower when the sight of the bud and the smell of its nectar will suffice to bring us into its presence without losing our own identity to the identity of the flower. The sacred aromatic odor of incense has the power to elevate the spirit, its pungent smoke invades the nostrils with its distinctive intensity and recreates for us in a sniff every temple, church or mosque we have ever visited. Scent should titillate, but not intoxicate, the centers of sensation, just as images should capture meaning and suggest significance without blinding the mind with flashes of light, without the defining distinctions of color to guide the way toward a sensible impression that is understandable and has meaning.

Odors are the advertisement of all they inhabit and serve; it is up to us to read the messages that they reveal to us. Borne on high by an invisible force, they reveal the wanderings of the wind even by their scents alone. Seafarers detect the richly scented bouquet of land-winds far at sea, while farmers who live close to the land can smell its sweet, earthy essence, and are attuned to the forces of nature by appreciating the fragrance of impending rain on the invisible currents of the north wind. The odor of earth within the plowed fields or the smell of semen emanating from freshly cut grass or the salty smell of the sea in the wind along the seashore all merge together with the smell of cut flowers and cooked spices and take their rightful place within the history of scent until we may hear them all chanting together in one grand anthem that rises to the heavens in a clear, primitive and wild vision that falls back to earth as a sweet remembrance of a higher order of reality. We are all earth-bound passengers on a journey of discovery, but we all travel the Milky Way together, men and women, scents on the wind, the trees of the forest and the flowers waving in the meadows, all travelers across distance and time in search of the meaning that every created thing is attempting to reveal. Many things and many journeys, some of them extensive, like the scent of the sea borne far inland by the wind or the warning of storm winds in the moisture of the air, all journeys of a sort that reveal unexpected destinations through sight and sound and scent, in sight of that distant Milky Way whose true destination reveals itself only at night to the inspired dreamer with a searching eye.

∾

We think that we smell with our noses, but that is a little like saying we hear with the wrinkled pouch of our ears. We can thank the olfactory organ[1] inside the nose for our ability to smell at all, not that we actually do the smelling with the hanging pouch of the nose. The human nose is an eloquent symbolic image of all that smelling entails. It gives structure, definition, and scope to the face in addition to being the front of an elaborate system of olfaction that is incredible to imagine, much less behold. What we take for granted would leave us devastated if the human visage were not supported by the articulation of a nose with which to smell the world and all its miraculous wonders. Only ask those people who are unable to smell the sensations of the world to find out what it means to be missing the blessing of this unique sense.

The nose actually plays front porch to an inner sanctum where specialized receptor cells of the olfactory epithelium detect and recognize smells. The air passes through the nasal cavity through a thick layer of mucous to the olfactory bulb. The smells are recognized there because each smell molecule fits into a nerve cell like the piece of a puzzle. The cells in turn send signals to the brain via the olfactory nerve. The brain then interprets those molecules as the sweet flowers or the sour milk that you've held up in your nose and

1. The olfactory region of each of the two nasal passages in humans is a small area of about 2.5 square centimeters containing in total approximately 50 million primary sensory receptor cells.

that produces a reaction of heaven and hell on your face. Each receptor is like a key on a typewriter, and each molecule types forth several letters to produce a word that signifies a particular odor. The descriptive "words" of the scent are then sent to the olfactory bulb, a pine nut-sized part of the brain right above the nose, where the words are turned into olfactory impressions that are distinctive and unique.

I don't intend to explain how cilia project themselves down from the olfactory epithelium into a pool of mucous that bathes the receptors with lipid-rich secretions that eventually become signals that reach the brain where they are interpreted as odors of an incredible variety of physical objects depending on their chemical constitution. It is enough of us to know that an incredible biochemical infrastructure exists behind the nose that supports and makes possible the ability to smell odors at all. The nose itself does nothing but serve as a symbolic image of the sense of smell, as well as the beloved instrument that serves the dark powers and the evocative mystery of scent.

&

In truth, every organic thing—and to some extent inorganic things as well—contain a unique scent and these scents orient human beings through distinctive and determining olfactory impressions that actually aid people in negotiating their way through the labyrinthine sensations of life. A distinctive odor remembers the memory of a loved one. The smell of a cigar immediately resurrects for me the image of my beloved father; burning leaves recalls my childhood memories of a New England autumn outside of Boston where I grew up, Jergens hand lotion summons the presence of my mother to my mind and heart as does the Jean Nate cologne that she loved. The intense odor of onions produces tears, while the stench of camembert cheese creates a sour face and a turned up nose. The power of a given scent initiates a multitude of impressions from remembrance to threat, from desire to repulsion. Aromas can elevate the spirit; they can lead us to our destination; they can warn us of an immanent threat; indeed as we shall soon elaborate upon, they can become a garland of higher consciousness whose rich bouquet serves in tribute to our origins and roots in the sweet remembrance of the Supreme Being who has created every living thing and Who makes a sublime unity out of the created universe.

The sacred images of revelation find their source in the Divine Word; but they also abound within the realm of nature and the kingdom of mankind. Adam is the composite image of the first primordial man, then the man fallen from grace, and thus the symbol *par excellence* of the perfectly human prototype man. The Hand of God summarizes in a word the miracle of the first creation and the instrument of all physical sensation and feeling. The heart is the abode of sacred sentiment and the seat of the intelligence. Rain is blessing; the wind is spirit; the night sky is the city of God, and scent is presence. While man is the greater symbol as well as a human revelation, the human senses of man are the lesser symbols of hidden truths that reveal far more than the impact of their intended outer functions in dealing with this world. Images of the senses conjure up a meaning that extends far beyond the literal image of the word. The eye represents intuitive vision and spiritual insight; the ear processes vibrations and reproduces sound; the hand recalls the act of creation in addition to the creativity of the arts and crafts. The images, symbols, words and narrative forms of revelation act as passageways or bridges into unfolding worlds of inner meaning and significance. They narrow the chasm that exists between visible and invisible worlds, between intelligible and incomprehensible realities, between outer and inner states of being. Ultimately, the revealed elements of the religion provide the formal channels of communication between beings of the human order and the Divine Being Himself.

In the Islamic tradition, elements of the natural order have deep symbolic value insofar as their image and essence escapes the physical form of the thing in order to introduce into the mind of the beholder an experience of a higher order of magnitude and a deeper level of spiritual remembrance. For example, the image of the vertical man is the image of the transcendent human being, the human alif, and the human prototype of *Homo spiritualis* who transcends the human form by virtue of his/her ability to know the idea of a Supreme Being, a Supreme Consciousness that substantiates the human consciousness and links this consciousness with the supreme manner of knowing, namely knowledge of the self.

In keeping with the traditional symbolic value inherent in the artefacts of the natural order, scent marks the identity of a presence, be it physical, corporeal, psychic or spiritual. We have already noted that all physical objects have a unique and distinctive scent that marks the very presence of the object. The blind can clearly identify a thing through its distinctive smell that can resemble no other thing. A rose is a rose and none other; just as the distinctive smell of the jasmine flower is unique as well as enveloping in its mystery and in its allure. Beyond physical objects, however, scent also has the power to signal a presence, whether it be ghostly, ethereal, or truly spiritual. We have all heard of the "cold wind" of the ghost and the "whisper" of the jinn, just as the creek of a door or the flutter of moth wings in the kiss of the moth bespeak of some dark secret too mysterious to reveal beyond the hint of a suggestion too ghostly to reveal. Many people have reported sensing the presence of close family members who have passed away by smelling suddenly the cigar of one beloved grandfather or the perfume of one's wife, an odor mingled with body chemistry of the loved one that is not only distinctive but also incomparable. It is interesting to speculate that if spirits on the other side wish for some reason to communicate with their still living earthly loves ones, they may attempt to do so through the evocative powers of scent, since their constitution resemble the structure if you will of ether and invisible odors trace their source to the ethereal world.

Scents have always played a major role in making connections with the spiritual world. The tombs of swamis, walis and saints often exude a peculiar odor that is attributed to the presence and spirit of the holy person as a lingering residue of their sacred presence, a reminder if you will of all that is sacred and holy with a power that is strong enough to resurrect sacred feelings within those visiting the tomb. I remember an unusual experience I had when visiting various places in Istanbul, Turkey. I found myself one afternoon looking past the grill into a mausoleum in which resided the tomb of Suleiman the Magnificent (1494–1566) alternatively known as the Lawgiver. Here was the greatest warrior of the

Ottoman empire who reigned for 46 years and extended the Ottoman empire to the gates of Vienna and as far West as Algeria in
North Africa. He presided over the Golden Age of the Ottoman
Empire during a time that represented the pinnacle of cultural
achievement in terms of architecture, literature, art, theology and
philosophy. I stumbled upon the tomb by accident one afternoon,
in back of the Suleimani Mosque in central Istanbul. The domed
mausoleum was grand enough in terms of design and architecture.
The tomb of the great sultan was raised on a dais and covered with a
green cloth inscribed with Quranic calligraphy with gold-embroi-
dered script. While I assumed that the tomb held some personage of
renown within its cold embrace, I had no idea it was the illustrious
Suleiman himself, the great 16th century monarch who was the rival
of King Henry the VIII of England and Ivan the IV of Russia, so-
called "the Terrible" (*Ivan Gronzy*)[2] until I read through my guide-
book and realized it was none other than the Magnificent himself.
There were a few other people milling about; but I had the grilled
window to myself through which you could see inside the mausoleum. In spite of the heat of the day, there was a cold and dusty chill
emanating from the enclosure of the tomb as I put my face to the
grill and the scent of dead leaves and mouldy wood assaulted my
nose with its aura of death and decay that even the Quranic calligraphy encircling the vaulted dome couldn't dissipate. Wherever the
soul of the great Suleiman had ended up, it certainly hasn't lingered
here in this neglected and abandoned burial place amid the shadows and cobwebs of a death that was truly eternal.

This experience stands in stark contrast to another tomb that I
took the opportunity of visiting just outside of Istanbul. It was not
easy to get to and required that I take several buses asking directions
along the way; but it was worth the effort on my part to find the
Ayyub Sultan Mosque situated outside the walls of Istanbul.[3] The

2. The term "terrible" in this instance being used in its archaic meaning of
"inspiring fear", rather than the modern day connotation of something terrible as
awful or horrible.
3. Built in 1458, it was the first mosque constructed by the Ottoman Turks following their conquest of Constantinople in 1453.

mosque rises on the spot where Abu Ayyub al-Ansare, the standard-bearer of the Prophet Mohammed, died during the Arab assault on Constantinople. His tomb is greatly venerated by Muslims and attracts many pilgrims throughout the year, although I didn't know that at the time. It was by accident that I found myself saying the mid-afternoon prayer in the mosque, the third ritual prayer of the day, at a time when the shadow of a man equals his height. After the prayer as I sat down to rest and refresh my soul by reading some Quran, I was befriended by several Turks who sat down on the floor in a circle around me and made their humble introductions. They were interested in my "story" and how I came to be sitting there in the mosque, an experience that is not uncommon for me being a Westerner and something of an anomaly sitting there cross-legged with the Quran spread open before me with its exotic script ornamenting the sun-faded pages, filling my eyes with its rhythmic lettering and my early with its harmonious and sacred sound vibrations. They simply cannot fathom this seemingly alien dream of a foreigner in their midst. It always seems to resurrect feelings of happiness and joy in the Muslims to learn the story of a person's conversion to their religion, as though someone had emerged from the depths of some ocean awash with the residue of its sparkling waters.[4] They told me that there was a *hadith* or traditional saying of the Prophet Mohammed which states that a Muslim convert is guaranteed the Paradise by virtue of this supreme act of conversion. I had heard this many times before, needless to say, and always feel humbled by these remarks and their generous attitude towards me. Before leaving to take their afternoon siesta, they told me about the tomb of Abu Ayyub on the other side of the courtyard within the mosque enclosure. I assured them that I would visit the tomb and make my traditional salaams to the beloved flag-bearer of the Prophet, after which they took their leave of me with respectful bows and a warm embrace.

I made my way over to the other side of the courtyard, opposite the central fountain where the worshippers could make their tradi-

---

4. See my book *Wisdom's Journey*, published by World Wisdom Books, Bloomington, Indiana, 2008.

tional ablutions before the ritual prayer, where I noticed a small domed building inlaid into the surrounding outer wall of the court-yard. There was a grill in the door of the small mausoleum and as I gazed into the dark interior, I was immediately struck by the sweet scent of some otherworldly odor that emanated from the tomb. The stone tomb itself rested in the interior of the circular room and was covered with a green gilded cloth and embellished with the elegant calligraphy of some Quranic verses. There is a strong tradition in Islam that identified scent with wind and spirit, the two Arabic *rih* and *ruh* are derived from the same root meaning. The Quran itself states that after Allah had fashioned the human being from water and clay, He "blew into him of His Spirit," thereby bringing the pri-mordial man Adam to life as the prototype first human being.

And spirit is none other than presence. When the brothers of Joseph brought back his shirt as proof to his bereaved father, Jacob, that his favorite son was still alive, the patriarch Jacob immediately smelt the "presence" of his beloved son, Joseph, in the shirt. When his brothers arrive home, Jacob said: "I do indeed scent the presence (*rih*) of Joseph." In its translated form, to "scent the presence" liter-ally means to feel the scent, air, atmosphere, even the breath of Joseph, for the word *rih* has all these implications and is a close derivative of the word spirit (*ruh*) in Arabic, the very same *ruh* that God breathed into the body of Adam. Needless to say, the beatific smells that unexpectedly flooded my sense of smell from the dark-ness of this tomb, in stark contract to the mouldy and dank chill of death that emanated from the tomb of Suleiman the Magnificent, lifted my mind and heart out of the doldrums of my routine day and sent me soaring upward as if in pursuit of birds in flight. The power of smell evokes higher levels of consciousness and experience that is quite simply undeniable, as much as we would like to deny the presence of God in our midst and live our lives as if He didn't exist.

I was suddenly struck out of my reverie in pursuit of the sublime, however, by the sound of footsteps. Two young men came up and stood beside me, attempting to peer through the grill into the inte-rior of the tomb. They both nodded and uttered the ritual salaam to me as I stood there on tiptoes looking into the dark interior. I noted that they were both strong, powerful looking men with a somewhat rough-edged demeanor and a little shabbily dressed. I remember thinking to myself, perhaps a little rudely, that I wouldn't want to meet these Turks in some dark alley under other circumstances. I politely stepped aside and gave way to their supplications to the saint buried within. I wondered briefly if they could smell what I did; but I didn't have to wait long for an answer to my rhetorical inquiry of mind. While one of them stood there and looked with interest into the enclave of the tomb, the other's face had reddened noticeably and he was holding both hands cupped in front of his face in a posture of grave supplication. At first, it is not something that I might have paid much attention to, and when I did notice something amiss, thought nothing of it until he suddenly began to sob quietly with a great heaving of his massive shoulders. I was stunned and looked with renewed interest into the depths of the tomb to see what he was seeing and had not noticed on my own. The other man began to comfort his friend, putting his hand over his shoulders and whispering soft Turkish phrases into his ear; but the friend would not be consoled and gave himself up completely to the emotion of the moment. He continued to utter profound sobs; as though he had some special insight that the world was about to end or that some grave personal misery was weighing unmercifully upon his shoulders.

A small wind blew around us as I felt myself caught up suddenly into the emotion of the moment. I looked into the tomb once again and thought of the great flag-bearer and companion of the Prophet whose remains lay within the enclosure and had done so for centuries; but what does the continuum of time matter in the face of an eternity of repose. The more the young man wept, the more I felt caught up suddenly in the spirit of the moment. The great hulk of a fellow now fell down on his knees and put his hands to the grill as though clinging for life. I myself began to weep, first innerly with a sinking of the heart and then real tears began to sprout from my eyes and down my cheeks as I surrendered to a moment that had suddenly and unexpectedly become irrevocably sacred. This was the so-called "gift of tears" of which the traditions speak, when, sparked by some unexpected catalyst, deep spiritual emotion comes to the surface of human consciousness with an overwhelming sense, first of a deep humility, followed then by profound awe in the face of some overwhelming reality, indeed the only reality that could ever matter to us mortals. It is an experience of high spiritual sentiment that actually induces real tears, in addition to the heart-felt sense of the sacred that we wish we could carry in the first tier of our consciousness everyday of our lives, but that we are grateful to have experienced for at least a few moments on rare occasions such as this. It is an act of purification followed by a radiant sense of bliss that is the inevitable result of some true realization of what condition we are in and what we have done or not done, followed by joy in the realization that there is a Supreme Being there to shed his blessing and light upon us and lead us to perfection that is the true vocation of humanity. The moment passed into eternity; but has lingered on some shelf of the mind to remind me of the sweet promise that life holds within its embrace and that sometimes finds its way into the tears of a raw emotion that ends up purifying the heart with the waters of its sweet revelation. Such is the unexpected experiences of the world. You enter a mosque to say a simple, ritual prayer in the mid-afternoon, and leave it later in the day a changed person with a shaken soul.

༄

In the grand mosque in Madinah, Saudi Arabia, I know I am nearing the tomb of the Prophet Mohammed through two clear pieces of evidence, the architectural change of the building which has a smaller, more crowded, and less grandiose aspect and dates back more than a millennium to the time of the Prophet and the early Caliphate era, and secondly by the density of the crowds of people all vying for proximity to the resting place of the Prophet. There is a section of the mosque cordoned off and positioned adjacent to the wall of the Prophet's tomb that is referred to and revered as the *al-riyadh al-jannah*, which roughly translates as "the garden of Paradise". The Prophet has referred to this part of the mosque by saying: "What is between my house and my minbar is a garden from the gardens of Paradise." It is an area that according to the traditions of the Prophet is actually a part of the Paradise that will rise upward and return to its original home on the Day of Judgment, which in Islam is alternatively referred to as the Day of Accounting (*yawn al-hisab*) and the Day of Religion (*yawn al-din*). Whatever the truth may be, I was soon to find out that this remarkable *riyadh* is certainly a place to sojourn for a while and rest because it provides an experience unique unto this world.

Many years ago when I first became Muslim and at a time several decades ago when the mosque was far less crowded than it is today, I remember quietly entering this section of the mosque and ensconcing myself cross-legged as is the custom on the light blue carpet distinguished from the red oriental carpets spread through the rest of the mosque. There was indeed not only a special quality of serenity and calm there that one would come to expect in the paradise, but I felt as I sat cross-legged and indrawn on the carpet as if I had come home at last and there was no where else I needed to go. An otherworldly fragrance seemed to unexpectedly permeate the air and I remember considering what that scent reminded me of until I had to confess that it reminded me of nothing related to this world, that it had an otherworldly quality that seemed exquisite and heavenly. Indeed the odor was paradisal.

The unexpected arrival of this rarefied aroma and its ethereal beauty bore a direct relation to the level of my consciousness, which seemed suddenly to take off on its own. As I sat in this "garden of Paradise", my mind took on wings and I began to soar higher and higher as a grand eagle in flight over lofty mountains. Call it auto suggestion of the tradition if you like, but a dream quality seemed to emerge like dawn mist over the waters of a lake. The strange, otherworldly scent began to raise my level of consciousness from the mundane to the sublime in some unconscious manner, and I felt I was entering another dimension virtually impossible to describe. Then, without warning, I felt a surge of emotion well up inside me from depths I didn't know existed, an emotive feeling so strong and satiating that I could do nothing but surrender to the power of these sacred emotions. I began to sob quietly with my head drawn down, the hot tears literally stream down my face and falling drop by drop only my kaftan. At first, the rational aspect of my mind clicked into gear as I actively wondered to myself why I was crying, even though I realized of course that the place, the moment, and the overall ambiance were strong enough to evoke such an unexpected, powerful reaction. The outburst was not convulsive or hectic; it was sheer weeping without an obvious catalyst. It was not the kind of grief that one experiences following the death of a loved one or the loss of a valued treasure; instead it was an emotive collapse without hill or valley, a release from the rigidity that holds us together in life, vast and inconsolable at first as a child's confrontation with some fleeting misery. The hot tears came as a soothing balm for the trials and tribulations of my life, the frustrations and the shattered hopes, the dreams, the remorse, the failures and even the valued successes that had come my way. I sobbed for the person I had been and the person I might well become. With time of course, the sobbing slowly died within me, throb by throb, until a wave as cool as spring water flowed across the shore of my being and an abiding peace streamed in rivulets through my mind and body. I had received the gift of tears spoken of in the traditions of Islam as a treasured spiritual experience in which the soul uses the mind and body to free itself of certain complexes of the psyche and the psychological knots of the spirit as a form of liberation from the lower self and as a means of self-purification. I eventually moved away from this area of the mosque, but not without leaving behind something of myself that didn't want to depart, a memory of the garden that beckons us from above while we live here below, a promise of revelation that I experienced for a few moments in the Prophet's mosque, in the black hills of Madinah, in a garden of the Paradise.

Similarly, at the Grand Mosque in Makkah, I had a unique experience that once again relates to the evocative power of scent. Whenever the Muslims enter the Haram, a central courtyard open to the heavens of grandiose proportion in which resides the Kaaba or house of Allah, they circumambulate the sacred cube seven times from right to left, commencing at a certain corner of the building in which is housed the celebrated sacred black stone (*hajar al-aswad*) that, according to apocryphal accounts, is a dark meteorite fallen down from the heavens. On one occasion, when I was making the *umrah* or minor pilgrimage,[5] I was accompanied by my Egyptian friend Amr, who promised to keep an eye on me and make sure that nothing improper happened as we performed the rites of the pilgrimage amid the chaos and confusion of the vast crowd.

With natural affection and an eagerness to accommodate, Amr took my arm and led me through the confusion of the crowd toward the swirling orbit of people moving about the Kaaba making invocations to Allah in a state of spiritual rapture. "We need to get as close to the Kaaba as possible," he whispered urgently in my ear. No sacramental dictate required us to get as close as possible to the house, yet custom and tradition suggested close proximity to the structure if at all possible and having made this once in a lifetime journey, all Muslims want to get as close to this symbolic edifice as possible. The Kaaba after all is a kind of proto-form of art whose spiritual dimension corresponds to myth or revelation and whose spiritual influence no Muslim wants to be far from, especially when so close to its actual presence. I also knew that Amr harbored a secret desire to kiss the black stone, and I confess so did I, said to be a meteorite fallen from Heaven that is lodged in a silver encasement in the east corner of the cubic structure and marks the place of commencement of the *tawwaf* or circumambulation.

No Muslim who has made *Hajj* or *Umrah* will deny that the circumambulation is a physical experience that takes stamina and will power. When you view the scene from the roof of the Grand Mosque or witness the event through TV cameras hoisted on high, it gives every appearance of being a rhythmic stream of humanity flowing in sublime unison around the central axis of the world. However, the reality of being amid this throbbing, densely packed mob is tumultuous and unpredictable and yet all the while nobody seems to care about the tumult around them or complain about the crush of people. Upon entering the throng, you loose your sense of personal identity and personal space and become one with a vast, teeming horde moving about the symbolic vision of the ancient

---

5. The *umrah* or minor pilgrimage can be performed in Makka at any time during the year. The *hajj* or formal pilgrimage, can be performed during a specific time period during the Islamic lunar month of *dhul Hajj.*

edifice and focusing all their hopes and aspirations on the reality of the Divine Being in a state of ecstatic rapture. It is like no experience in "this world" and virtually takes the worshippers well beyond the threshold of their daily consciousness into realms of experience they have never experienced before and may never experience again, at least in this world.

Entering the ritual practice of circumambulation is like entering into the "one upon a time" of myths and folktales, *in illo tempore*. The pilgrim enters into sacred time that is actually the "real" time of the "vertical" or eternal dimension, as opposed to the horizontal, linear and progressive time that we experience here on earth as a relentless, forward-moving machine that propels us seemingly forward, as if forward is the only place we need to go. I fell immediate victim to this sublime transcendent state of mind as if by some remote control of heaven and felt at one with the rotating vortex of the crowd. I no longer seemed to matter as an individual entity for I had been swept away in this "first sanctuary", according to the traditions, to a primordial time of perfection and heightened consciousness when the truth is there to behold, there to witness, and there to be known as nothing else can be known. As I circumambulate the sacred Kaaba, I make my entreaties, I send my greetings, I pray to Allah and worship the Divinity. Soon enough, beyond all reckoning of time, I am truly swept away by a flood of emotion and higher sentiment as I become one with the wave of worshippers. Indeed, I feel myself giving up and surrendering to this moment of eternity in time and this central place that makes possible the ascent of humanity beyond the horizon of the rational mind and beyond the dictates of the lower self.

Amr has managed to seize a seven beaded cord resting on the wall by the Station of Ismael along one side of the Kaaba with which to keep track of the seven circumambulations that are required of the *tawwaf* ritual, although how he has managed this feat is anyone's guess as he grins sheepishly at me holding aloft the beaded cord. Our arms are locked together for security as we make our way round after round within the circumference of the sacred precinct. I am happy to have this beloved person with me, who forever after will be a friend in spirit, as we make the circumambulation in communion with the Spirit of God that overshadows the environment with its blessed grace. It feels as though I have known my friend Amr for a thousand years.

Perhaps it is the writer and natural-born observer in my nature, but I unconsciously take the time to notice the behavior and movement of the people around me. Everyone seems solicitous of the other's safety and comfort, although admittedly the movement around the Kaaba is far from harmonious at ground zero. It takes effort just to keep standing and one is literally carried forward on tiptoes by the mob pressing in on every side. Still, no one exaggerates the hectic quality of the procession and everyone seems to be trying to defer to the person nearby out of respect for the moment. Of course, there is every size, shape, and color of person to be imagined in this vast horde of humanity. I see the elderly and the young, husbands and wives, fathers, sons and daughters. There are groups of women clinging together for safely and surprisingly strong as they race past me. There are groups of men, from Iran, from Ethiopia, from Malaysia, from China, arms linked together in a chain for support. People of all races and nationalities are praying aloud, uttering in Arabic the Quranic epithets and litanies that are appropriately noted for the occasion, entreaties to Allah for health, for blessing, for provision, for the *hasanat* or good things of this and the next world. The elderly and the crippled are being carried in litters overhead on the hands of husky black Africans; others are being moved along in wheelchairs by family members or friends. In one shocking instance, I felt a rustle at my feet and upon looking down toward the marble floor of the enclosure, I see to my horror amid the disorder of moving legs a crippled woman crawling along in circumambulation on all fours with a look of determination and joy spread across her face.

I cling to my Egyptian friend Amr for stamina and support, approaching an age when I can call myself elderly and fearful of falling down and being overrun by this juggernaut of moving humanity. On the sixth round, a way close to the wall of the Kaaba suddenly opens, seemingly miraculously, for both Amr and I noticed that the agitated waters of humanity that enclosed us have unexpectedly opened a path to give free passage to the vicinity of the *Hajar al-Aswad*, the black stone. I think to myself that the intentions of Amr and I are of one accord as he jerks my arms and drags me sideways through the throng toward the sacred stone.

Under normal circumstances, it is well nigh impossible to get anywhere near this sacred artifact for the crowds that are clambering to touch and kiss the holy object. Amr suddenly saw the opportunity and made his move, veering toward the black stone and dragging me alongside with him. We were immediately engulfed once again by the teeming throng of people surrounding the stone and only footsteps away from touching the sacred object. I looked up and saw Amr standing by the silver frame of the black stone grinning broadly with satisfaction. I knew that he had achieved his goal and had touched the stone. I tried to lean forward and had my arm extended as far as possible in the direction of the blessed object, but I simply could not move another inch forward. I was about to give up the effort and blend back into the human wave, when I felt a hand seize my wrist and move it down into the framed enclosure wherein resides the *Hajar al-Aswad*. It is the swift movement of Amr's powerful grip that has made this possible. For a brief moment, I feel the cool, electrifying presence of the stone run up through my arm and down into my soul and I smell the unearthly fragrance of the Paradise evoking a memory of some primal purity and perfection amid the chaos of the moment. Then, we were both summarily thrown beyond the area of the building containing the black stone by the crowd surging forward around the corner, whence we raise our right hands to greet the Divinity one last time before commencing the final *tawwaf* around the Kaaba.

Once again, the senses of smell and touch reveal the essence of their own inner experience, taking people places they never thought they would venture and offering them an open door to the sublime world of higher spiritual experience they never thought would happen through direct contact with the physical world. Yet, having reached out, passed through, and been lifted up beyond the shelf of some inner horizon you never knew existed, you can only gaze in wonder at the mysteries that suddenly reveal themselves, making available to the unsuspecting mind an understanding that the senses are far more than signposts and instruments in the verification of a purely physical reality. They literally have the power to open a door to the Infinite.

◠

Finally, the sense of smell plays a major role among the faithful in Islamic countries as an aid in the remembrance of God when performing their religious duties. Oftentimes, the Muslims experience waves of an exquisite, otherworldly aroma emanating from the holy book as they sit and read the Quran after prayer, for recitation of the Quran in Islam is a form of worship in Islam in the same way that prayer is a form of worship. This is perhaps not that surprising when the traditional sources themselves suggest that the Quran in some mysterious manner contains the perfume of the soul of the person through whom it was revealed. Since the revelation literally passed through the mind and soul of the beloved Prophet, it is small wonder that the book itself may sometimes give off a beatific scent that remembers the Prophet who delivered the divine revelation to humanity. It is not uncommon for Muslims to sit down on their prayer carpets either before or after the early morning prayer to read and recite the Holy Quran. The pale rays of the waning moon may lay across the window sill. In the pre-dawn darkness, the stars twinkle their message of the eternity of time, while the panorama of the night sky itself makes its bold statement of the infinitude of form, as endless in its physical projection as it is mysterious to the rational mind. There is a hint of incense and musk in the air which capture an inner meaning that is capable of subtly influencing the mind and spirit of the reader of the holy text of the revelation. Heavenly scents accompany the two angels who descend to witness the Quranic recitation that occurs in one place or another every morning across the far crescent of the Islamic world.

Both incense and perfume create a particular atmosphere through sheer smell that is generally associated with the spiritual practices of the religion. Certainly incense has traditionally been considered the world over as a spiritual support to various forms of worship across the spectrum of the religions, although it is also used as a prescription in medicine and as a cultural artefact with aesthetic qualities for raising people's spirits.[6] Frankincense[7] and myrrh[8] were the ceremonial and symbolic gifts of the Magi because of their close association with their power to create through these unique natural substances a spiritual ambiance. Myrrh was especially used in ancient times because of its medicinal properties. In Chinese medicine, it is used to increase heart rate and circulation and as a liniment for bruises, aches and sprains. Incense has been used traditionally down through the centuries in mosques, churches and temples for religious rituals, to create an ambience that relates directly to smell, refreshing the mind and body with the outer sense of smell, but innerly refreshing the entire breath/spirit of the individual with its immediate and direct associations with the realm of the spirit. Muslims often fuse thick clouds of incense into their beards and turbans and it is considered an honor to be offered the balm of smoky incense into one's clothing after a meal, especially during the holy month of Ramadhan.

Musk is identified in the Quran as a scent of the Paradise[9] and is traditionally applied to the body, especially the hands, beard and head, before the prayer in Muslim countries. Together with incense, musk is often used to enhance, through the sense of smell, the inner

6. Incense is derived from compounds within the natural order, including such categories of plant life as woods and barks (cedar, sandlewood and juniper), seeds and fruits (star anise, nutmeg, coriander and vanilla), resins and gums (frankincense, myrrh and camphor), leaves (patchouli, sage, bay and tea), and finally flowers and buds (clove, lavender, saffron).

7. The name itself comes from the "incense of the Franks" because it was introduced into Europe by Frankish Crusaders. The resin is also knows as *olibanum* (from the Arabic *al-luban* roughly translated as "that resulting from milking", referring to the milky sap from the tree Boswellia. The lost city of Ubar in Oman is said to have been the center of the frankincense trade in ancient times.

8. Like frankincense, myrrh is the dried sap of an ancient tree, *Cammiphora myrrha* located in Somalia and eastern Ethiopia. Myrrh was used as an embalming ointment and as a penitential incense in funerals and cremations. It is said that the Roman Emperor Nero burned a year's worth of myrrh at the funeral of his wife, Poppaea.

9. They are given to drink of a pure wine, sealed; the seal thereof will be musk, for this let all those strive who strive for bliss (Quran 83:25–26). When asked what he favored most by his companions, the Prophet Mohammed included scent, together with prayer and women, as the three most favored things in "this world".

experience provided by the prayer. The profound and penetrating scents of musk and incense remind Muslims of their divine connections and serve as direct remembrances (*dhikr*) of God. So powerful is the association of these holy smells with the Islamic prayer ritual that the very smell of these odors in the passing wind is enough to remind the faithful of their spiritual and religious duties. In this way, the outer forms of the senses possess psycho-spiritual properties that can lead the mentality of an individual beyond mere forms in the direction of the celestial realities that lie at the heart of all forms. It is not surprising that aromatherapy has begun to take hold of the imagination of many people within modern societies today as an alternative therapy to depression and sickness, a therapy that has long been the mainstay of traditional societies who knew the value of sacred smells and used these smells not only to ward off temptation and misery, but also to raise their consciousness and enhance their spirits with the spirits of these enriching and evocative scents.

How infinitely superior to our physical senses are those of the inward senses that flow from body to mind to soul to spirit in the same manner that birds fly through clouds and over mountain peaks, upheld by the force of the spirit in defiance of the force of gravity and the laws of the natural order. Flowers have been admired down through the millennia for their color and form, but it is the scent of the lilac and the rose that sends our spirits aloft with their sublime olfactory essence. We see the flower and feel pleasure at its sight, but to smell the unique beauty of its essence is to be enfolded within its rich mystery and in the beauty of its implicit harmony. The smoke of burning incense rises in the air in florid arabesques, creating fingers and curlicues in slow motion that literally float like clouds and form a virtual calligraphy of scent that punctuates the air with its hypnotic presence before entering the nose with its holy, evocative aroma until finally arriving within the sacred niches and deep grottoes within the mind and heart.

The value of these smells lies in their ability to remind us of our supernatural origins. The exotic aroma of flowers and the wild smells that lie secreted in the texture of woods, leaves and resins come to the attention of our sense of smell to remind us of something that we have perhaps forgotten. These odors that arise from the natural order are always nearer to their origin than we can imagine and their origin is in perfect harmony with the Origin of all things. Even the evanescence of flowers is not a matter for regret; on the contrary it is an ever-present reminder of who we are and what we need to remember. These essences remind us of our supernatural origins and serve as a kind of guarantee of the immutability of the qualities that lie within them that so delight us and lift our spirits toward the remembrance of our own true origins. The Buddha was sitting with his disciplines who had assembled to hear him preach a sermon; but he said not a word. Instead, he stooped down and plucked a flower and held it up for them to see. Of all the assembly, only one showed by his smile that he understood the Buddha's message. In the company of a rose, words of explanation are not necessary.

The evocative sense of smell serves humanity as an instrument of realization and possibly of transcendence. Whether they be the pine resins and saps of the primordial forests and the salty broth of the global oceans, or the perfumes and incense within the sacred domain of the natural order, or the hint of a presence in the lingering scent of a cloth or a kerchief that whispers of some higher, other-worldly spirit making itself known in the only way it has available, scents make their inevitable way beyond the physical form to a higher plane of experience through the human sense of smell. The mysterious power of scent evokes the experience of a reality that can be experienced directly and intuitively, just as beauty and truth are apprehended directly and intuitively, rather than through the analytical and imaginative power of the mind alone, much less through some mathematical formula. The direct apprehension of the reality lies prefigured in the natural and unaffected delight that lies within the scents and smells of the flower and tree and leaf. These essential odors become the grand wings that sweep us along the broad concourse of life in experiencing the physical world, lending us the lift to flow over chimneys and rooftops, across vast oceans and rolling savannahs, over great mountain peaks and deep into the canyons of the earth to reveal the images and sounds and scents of an abiding destiny. In so doing, are placed on the arrow of God, riding fast and sure through the peaks and valleys of life, in the certitude of His Reality and the unity of His abiding truth that there is only one God but He.

4

THE RESONATING
POWER OF SOUND

Heard melodies are sweet,
but those unheard are sweeter. (Keats)

Could we live without the sweet scent of the lilac or the pungency of sage and still attain the paradise? No doubt. Could we pass through life without the benefit of sight and the glorious visions the world has to offer? Perhaps, because many blind people are undoubtedly in heaven. Could we forfeit our ability to taste the culinary delights on offer at the dinner table? Undoubtedly, although not without regret. Could we forgo the sound of the voices that every created thing gives utterance to and accept the silence that only outer space has to offer? The answer lies with those deaf mutes that pass through life in the profound silence of a soundless world.

When we think of the five human senses, we think of them in terms of what they have to offer. When we wish to appreciate their vital connection with our lives, for example, we need only think of what it would be like without the sight of our eyes or the music of our ears or the delectable smells and taste on offer to human connoisseurs by the sublime temptations of food. What we could not live effectively without and still attain the paradise is the perceptions of the inner eye, the aromatic smells of every created thing that warn us of their true essence, the listening that transcends sheer sound in lifting the human spirit beyond earthly realms, the taste of an experience that opens a secret door to the other side of reality, the ability to channel the inner world of sentiment and emotion through the sense of touch in connecting us with the world. All of the inner senses reclaim the intuitions and insights that the outer senses have given up in their superficial allegiance to the physical world, pretending that what they see, hear, taste, touch and smell represents the only reality that exists and that we humans need to surrender to.

There exists a natural tension between silence and sound that highlights a similar tension that exists between the cacophony of the world and the silence of the celestial spheres. We live in a world of sound to the extent that virtually every created thing both animate and inanimate has a voice that gives something of their essence away and portends their true nature. What complements the true nature of this world and all its physical forms refer back to archetypes and serve as symbols—whether through image, gesture, or sound—of a higher reality of the spiritual world that transcends the physical plane of existence. The song of the lark and the call of the peacock are distinctive and unique to these animals and summarizes through sound something of their essence. The lilting beauty of the lark in stark contrast to the melancholy cry of the peacock represents an experience that only highlights the unique nature of these animals. Trees rustle in the wind; hinges creek on their doorframe; the drum resounds; the bell resonates. Cicadas hiding in trees create a stampede of sound that characterizes the essence of a long, hot, summer afternoon. Frogs chirp their distinctive burp in the darkness of country swamps. Thunder complements lightning while lightning itself is the silent, fiery sword of heaven, taming the earth and terrorizing everyone who inhabits it with grand displays of light streaking across the heavens as though the sky itself were but a pond to reflect the spectacular display of God's power. Both thunder and lightning, as artifacts of silence and sound, terrorize the world with their magnificent show of sound and light and their dramatic effect resonates on our ear and mind as a reflection of something otherworldly and beyond the horizon of this world.

The ear itself is a miraculous instrument of reception and grace that always operates in pairs and ultimately connects within the cranium through its labyrinthine, auricular canals to provide the brain with a focused sense of sound. It is interesting to note that all the senses have decorative as well as functional instruments that serve as windows of the mind as well as the outer symbol of an inner experience. Although the ear is the vertebrate sense organ that recognizes sound, it is the brain and central nervous system that "hears". Sound begins of course with movement, any movement at all within the physical framework of the world. It is an onrushing, cresting and subsiding wave of air molecules that float out from the movement as though with a life of its own and a justification in its own pure existence. The waves of sound roll into our ears like a surging tide of water that sets the eardrum vibrating, setting in movement the three smallest bones in the body, appropriately named the hammer, the anvil, and the stirrup. Sound waves are perceived by the brain through the firing of nerve cells in the auditory portion of the central nervous system. The ear changes sound pressure waves from the outside world into a signal of nerve impulses sent to the brain. When sound strikes the ear drum, the movement is transferred to the footplate of the stapes, which presses into one of the fluid-filled ducts of the cochlea. The fluid inside this duct is moved, flowing against the receptor cells of the organ of Corti, which fire, thus transforming sound waves into nerve impulses, sending information through the auditory portion of the eighth cranial nerve to the brain. Lo and behold, we hear.

The question is: Are we listening? After all, it is possible to hear something without actively engaging the substance of the sound. Isn't that why we distinguish people who are good "listeners" from people who pretend to hear, but who do not actively listen to the import of the communication? Sound management strategists now consider the skills of listening and of being a good listener to be crucial in the effective interaction between management and their human resources. I once had a close friend who was an audiophile. He spent thousands of dollars on state of the art electro-static speakers that were elegant in shape and resembled Chinese room dividers. He played all the great classics from Bach to Wagner and was an astute opera lover, having the ability to recognize a singer's voice within seconds of listening to it. However, I came to the conclusion after years knowing him and observing his obsession with his speakers and the audio support system that fed the sound to the speakers, that he never actually listened to the music. He was too busy listening to the "quality" of the sound and moving the speakers around the room for supposedly optimum effect.

We think of sound as pitch, intonation, and echo within a certain order of magnitude because we are earth-bound creatures and can only truly appreciate the dimension that we inhabit. After all, the order of magnitude of outer space represents an eternity of time and infinity of space that is quite simply incomprehensible to the human mind. Although the horizon is always there as the hem of the earth wherever we turn and the proto-symbol of the mystery that lies beyond its proverbial edge, it is as nothing in its order of magnitude in comparison with the vast scope of the universe set forth as a metacosmic, symbolic image in the night sky. Beyond its capacity as levels of noise, and beyond its technical aspect as reso-nance translated into nerve impulses of the brain, and beyond its function that identifies objects and permits us to take part in the daily commerce of the world, sound contains the crucial thread that connects us to the physical world. We rely on sound not only to ele-vate our spirits and enliven our sensibilities, we depend on sounds to help us interpret, communicate with, and express our impres-sions of the world around us.

☙

There is no doubt that there are objects and instruments in the world that establish resonant cadences that directly affect the human sensibility and touch the human heart with their infecting and melancholy sound. The eerie melody of a distant horn evokes feelings of longing and loss as its reverberations make their way over the edge of some distant horizon to reach our expectant ears with its evocative music. The distinctive sound of a distant train passing through the valleys of the night evokes feelings of travel and destination, time passing and people on their way to places we have never been. The intoning of a church bell across the rooftops of a pastoral village resurrects feelings of reverence and praise that lie sequestered within our beings as a remembrance of the golden age of the primordial era when humanity had direct perception of the other side of reality and never questioned the possibility of the world of the spirit as the true counterpoint to the physical reality that we presently worship today as the only reality. The sounding of the church bell contains its own prayer, in addition to the prayers that rise up from the parishioners within the church, sending its solemn resonance through the air and into human ears as a faint reminder of their true nature and place within the design of the universe. We readily respond to the sound of some distant bell because we contain within ourselves an inner bell that when intoned sends reverberations deep in the ground of the human soul with its message of harmony and truth. The rhythmic percussion of a drum, generated by a taut skin membrane spread tightly across a piece of wood, sends waves through the ground, up through the feet, and into the heart of the listener with its intense pulsating beat, in frank imitation of the beating of the human heart. Drums are used for percussion and setting the pace for musical melodies, but they have also been used down through history as a form of communication. The tribes of Africa were adept at using talking drums for communication in the same manner that the Red Indians of North America used smoke signals to communicate effectively with their comrades across vast distances between mountain peaks.

In addition, pure sound evolved into sacred sound for traditional peoples down through history. If we wish to understand the profound repository of spiritual practices that traditional people had available to them in earlier time periods, it is necessary to reflect firstly upon the single, most important factor that underlies all rites and rituals, namely the magic and power of words through sound, indeed through sacred sounds, that enliven and substantiate all prayer, meditation, invocation, incantations, scripture reading, mantras, and recitation of all sacred formulas and epithets. Modern humanity cannot even imagine how profoundly the so-called pagan, primitive man experienced the magic of sheer sound, words, and speech. We cannot imagine, for example, to what degree and depth the enormous influence certain sounds had on the culture and the way of life of earlier civilizations, especially in the religious aspects of those societies and how they expressed themselves spiritually through sacred words and phrases. We cannot imagine it simply because we no longer believe in the implicit power of sound and we no longer value the efficacy of the sacred word. The power of sound and the efficacy of the revealed word could continue to have a purpose and a meaning for modernite individuals, if only they had the imagination and the inclination to listen and feel the hidden power contained within the sacred and primordial vibrations of certain words and sounds.

The value and power of sound, its secrets and its latent magical forces, had been well understood by the seers, shamans, and practitioners of former, more traditional times. The Rishis who inhabited the slopes of the Himalayas, the Magi of Iran, the adepts of Mesopotamia, the priests of Egypt, and the philosophers of Greece and the mystics of the Arab world, all understood and used the power of sound in their spiritual practices in order to establish a rhythm and a vibration through chanting, incantations and music that transcended the literal word in order to penetrate into the mysterious and magical forces that actually form the key to the riddles of creation and creativeness, while at the same time revealing something about the nature of things and of the phenomena of life. Pythagoras, an initiate of Eastern wisdom and a founder of one of the most influential schools of mystic philosophy in the West, spoke of the "harmony of the spheres" in which every created thing down to the atom produced a particular sound because of its movement and its rhythm, creating a vibration that was unique unto itself. The idea of a creative sound was perpetuated through the teachings of the divine *logos*[1]. The tradition and knowledge of the creative sound lived on in India through various Yoga-systems, found refinement in the Schools of Buddhism, and has been preserved in theory as well as in practice, in the countries of Mahayana Buddhism from Tibet to Japan.

In fact, the absolute use of sound makes its first appearance at the time of primordial dawn, when the Divinity desired to be made

---

1. The gospel of St. John commences with the mysterious words: "In the beginning was the Word, and the Word was with God, and the Word was God, and the Word was made flesh."

manifest, remembering the traditional saying in Islam that reports the Divine Being saying in a *hadith qudsi*: "I was a hidden treasure and I wanted to be known. Therefore I created the world." In exploring the meaning and characterizing the forms of worship that were available to traditional man, and that still could be made available to modern man, we need to return for a moment to the prelude and dawn of the primordial wilderness and listen! The inaudible was made audible, the invisible was made visible, and the intangible was made tangible. According to the Quran, nothingness emerged out of itself to become a manifested something through the utterance of the sound word BE (*KUN*). The sacred Quranic revelation relates that the act of creation commenced with a sacred sound: "Be (*kun*) and it immediately becomes" (*fa yakoon*) (19:35). All of creation, including the very act of creation, can be reduced to the sacred sound of a primordial utterance, a cosmic sound that translates into the creation and manifestation of the visible word. In this way, the Divine Being was "a hidden treasure" that became manifest.

Thereafter, what distinguished the primordial or golden era and the primordial generations who peopled that era, with Adam as the symbolic first man, was the fact that Adam was given the power of the sacred word from the Divine Being. The Quran tells us that Adam was taught "the names of things" and therefore he was able to distinguish himself from the angels and the animals because of the inherent power he enjoyed to communicate through sound symbols and words the essence of things. For Adam and subsequent generations, speech was sacred and symbolic. In other words, sound conveyed a meaningful knowledge, and the accumulated sound representations signified knowledge to be experienced behind the images. The human being as personified through Adam could consciously think, identify, know and give voice through vibratory and distinctive sound to the essence of things. This ability represented tremendous power and tremendous prescience. It was tantamount to being able to articulate the full creative scope of his mind as well as the meaning of the world through its exploration and discovery. The secret of the act of creation and the secret of the creative word has come together into a sacred alliance in order for humanity to express the true meaning of life as we experience it without filters or barriers.

When Adam was given the names of things, he actually took possession of the world and became, as the Quran relates, the *khalifah Allah* or God's representative on earth, to rule over his appointed domain, so long as he surrendered his will to the absolute Will of the Divinity. By way of compensation, humanity discovered a new dimension, a world within themselves, opening upon the vista of a higher consciousness and a higher expression of life beyond the existing condition of humanity, a condition that is foretold in the bliss of the paradise, bliss that remembers and recreates the plenitude of the primordial era. It represented inner experience that goes beyond the senses and can be initiated through vibration, sound, rhythm and ultimately a melody of the spirit that through prayer and the other spiritual practices ultimately leads to fulfilment of the soul and transcendence of the spirit.

The revelation portrays divine sound as having initiated the movement, rhythm and harmony of the universe. Therefore, it is not as farfetched as it may first seem to the modern mentality that, through sound, humanity will once again find the possibility of fine-tuning themselves with the spiritual vibrations that are in the very nature of things and strike the holy cord that is in the very nature of the human being. Both ancient and modern scriptures suggest that the creative act in its first step towards manifestation was audible, followed by the visible, and ultimately the tangible signs of the universe.

Even modern science has discovered that sounds actually create impressions that can be made visible. We have only to think of both the physical and mental effects that sound has on the human entity to realize that a spiritual effect also exists as a potential force within man. The roll of thunder can raise the hair on the back of the arm and head; a shout can cause goose bumps on the body; a scream has the power to curdle blood. A whisper can tempt, enthral, soothe, convey secrets or create intimacy. A soulful cry can create fear, terror, sadness, joy, even spiritual ecstasy, while the human sigh can reflect sorrow, satisfaction, frustration, exhaustion, and resignation. There is, when you explore the possibilities, a limitless capacity of sounds to create "states or stations" of experience that reach deep into the interior of the human being, and into the deep stream of life itself, through the mysterious power of sound.[2]

ॱ

All that is visible, clings to the invisible,
the audible to the inaudible,
the tangible to the intangible:
Perhaps the thinkable to the unthinkable.
(Novalis)

At some remote dawn of pre-history, sound evolved to become word. Meaning evolved into communication. The primordial word became letters, words, images, symbols and ultimately names that set the stage for a universal *Ursprache* or proto-language that constituted the formative principle of all communication in this world. For the unmanifested, inner world of spirit, the sound/word became a *mantra*,[3] a spiritual formula, or the Name of Names, in order to serve humanity as a consciousness-raising instrument of the mind and a spiritual vehicle of mysterious forces to connect humanity with the inaudible, invisible, and even the unthinkable.

The invocation of the Name is a method that cuts across a number of religious traditions including Buddhism, Christianity, and Islam, all of which recommend both silent and oral remembrance (*dhikr*) of the Supreme Name of the given tradition. In Japanese Amidic Buddhism, there is a method of meditation that is associated with the school of Jodo or "Pure Lane" in which the name of

2. Snake charmers, found mostly in India, but also in other parts of the world such as in Marrakech, Morocco, play their *pungi*, a simple wind instrument in order to attract cobras and other snakes from the vicinity. The cobra seems to forget the instinct to protect itself from the attack of man or other creatures. The cobra begins to raise its head and move it right and left. As long as the eerie melody of the instrument is played, the cobra remains mesmerized and continues to move to and fro in a kind of ecstasy, impervious to the outside world.

3. In the word *mantra*, the root *man* = "to think" (in Greek *menos*, in Latin *mens*) is combined with the element *tra*, which forms tool words. Thus, mantra is a tool for thinking, a "thing which creates a mental picture."

Buddha Amitabha, meaning "Infinite Light", is invoked in order for the postulates to connect their mind and heart with the higher realities implicit in the Name. In Tibetan Buddhism, the six syllable phrase OM MANI PADME HUM, has been described as "the quintessence of the wisdom of all the Buddhas." In Christianity, the quintessential formula is the Jesus Prayer, which is associated generally with the churches of the Eastern Rite. This prayer is a well-known and well-practised spiritual method that goes under the name of Hesychasm, which comes from the Greek word *hesychia*, meaning "tranquillity".[4] Finally the continued remembrance (*dhikr*) of the Name of Allah, whether silently or orally, brings about the "divine encounter" of the human heart with the Spirit of God, and no other encounter could be more profound or more sublime from the Islamic point of view than this.

Mantras are audible sounds of visual symbolic representations. They are employed in Buddhist ritual as instruments of the mind and/or vehicles for the enhancement of the spirit. Mantras, the most famous being the Buddhist OM MANI PADME HUM,[5] are an extremely complex and sensitive subject matter whose full significance and import cannot be explain in a few paragraphs. It is worth pointing out in the context we are now discussing, however, that the power and implications of the sacred word is accepted within a number of spiritual traditions. The mantra has broad implications as a spiritual instrument that forms the basis and conceptualization

4. The monastic centers in Russia and the Balkan countries had eminent masters, called *geron* in Greek and *staretz* in Russian. The "Elder" Zosima, in Dostoevski's *Brothers Karamazov*, is an imaginative portrait of such a master. Mont Athos is the most famous center where these methods were—and still are—practised; but they are also traced back to the Desert Fathers in Egypt and other parts of the Christian East. The Jesus Prayer, made famous in the 19th century spiritual tract *The Way of the Pilgrim*, R.M. French (tr.), Harper SanFrancisco, 1991, reads as follows in Latin: *Domine Jesu Christe Fili Dei miserere nobis*, in English "Lord Jesus Christ, Son of God, have mercy on me."

5. For a complete presentation and analysis of the esoteric principles that lie behind this world famous mantra and the underlying philosophy of Tibetan Buddhism, see Lama Govinda's *Foundations of Tibetan Mysticism* (York Beach, ME, Sam Weiser Inc., 1991). The work is regarded as a classic of Tibetan mysticism and clearly and fully explains the esoteric principles of the mantra.

for a number of spiritual disciplines and practices in Buddhism and whose implications spread across the entire traditional landscape. The mantra is not only a form of speech, it is also a form of power. When the sound of the mantra is expressed, it enters the world as a reality and something "happens". The vibration that it establishes becomes a rhythm and a harmony. In this sense, a mantra is a deed rather than a word or group of words, acting immediately on the individual, and by extension it moves through him out into the universal cosmos.

We are now living in the age of multi-media. Our age is a time characterized by the free flow of information through vast computer networks, such as the Internet, with its capacity to instantaneously connect people world-wide. The spoken and written word has been multiplied a million fold or even a billion fold. Words and ideas are indiscriminately thrown at the mass population in ways that the public has never dreamed of before. Possibilities are becoming apparent through fast advancing technological developments with the computer and its increasing interdependence on other forms of communication such as telephone and television to the extent that most technocrats developing these things still don't know how and to what end these technological advances can best be utilized by the public. However, one effect is obvious. The value of the word as such has reached such a low standard that it is difficult to give even a faint idea of the reverence with which people of more spiritual times or more religiously orientated civilizations approached the word, the mantra, the prayer, or the invocation of the holy Name of Names. To traditional man, sacred words in a variety of forms were considered vehicles of a hallowed tradition and the very embodiment of the Holy Spirit.

From the spiritual perspective, certain sounds precede language insofar as language is understood to convey a specific meaning. Mantras precede language and go far beyond language as such in its normal conceptualization and usage. It may be an archetypal sound which does not obey any rule of how to form words. In addition, the mantra reveals meaning that goes far beyond the literal explanations of words. Like music, it has significance and a meaningfulness that cannot be expressed or limited to mere words. In the same way that music has an inner significance and an profound meaning established through vibration, rhythm, and ultimately melody that cannot be expressed in words, so also the mantra has a deep inner significance and an unfathomable meaning on different levels which can only be understood through usage and practice, thus transforming the mantra from a theoretical insight into a spiritual experience.

For example, no one can tell precisely what a sound like OM or HUM means because its meaning reaches beyond the human domain into the cosmic realm. In fact, the sound/word OM is used differently in Buddhism and Hinduism. In Hinduism, this ancient and hauntingly beautiful sound was used in a somewhat non-specific manner either at the beginning of a mantra, at its end, or at any other location within the mantra utterance. In Buddhism, however, it has a specified and clearly defined place. OM can be used only at the beginning of a combined mantra such as OM MANI PADME HUM, while HUM can be used only at the end of the mantra. OM always precedes a combined mantra and HUM closes it. "The OM stands for the all-inclusive universal level, whereas HUM leads into the depth of our own heart or, to put it differently, moves from the universal level down to the level of the individual. This is because we can experience the universal only as an individual. Individuality is therefore as important as universality."[6] In a manner of speaking, we can say that the sound/word OM therefore reaches down from the universal cosmic experience to enter the human domain, while HUM reaches up from the depths of the human heart in order to meet this cosmic sound, thus making possible the realization of the universal and the individual within the human being in a meeting most profound.

OM MANI PADME HUM is what is called a combined mantra. OM and HUM are *bijas* or seed mantras, the two words between OM and HUM can be translated because the words MANI and PADME have a meaning or perhaps one should write various meanings on different levels of expression. Literally translated

6. Lama Govinda, *Insights of a Himalayan Pilgrim* (Berkeley, CA: Dharma Publishing, 1991), p. 163.

MANI PADME means the "jewel in the lotus flower." Who is the jewel? The jewel is of course the Buddha, Dharma, and Sangha. Here we can connect the word/symbol jewel with a meaning which transcends the meaning associated with a precious stone. On the other hand, the precious jewel is also the Buddha as embodiment of realized enlightenment. PADME stands for our spiritual center, our "heart". Grammatically, PADME is locative, meaning "within the lotus flower," i.e., within the heart, or the innermost spiritual center of the human being.

The use of mantras, however, is no mere theoretical and abstract projection of spiritual possibility. They are used in real life in Buddhist lands, most notably in a country such as Tibet. The Chinese may have overrun the land and destroyed the external artefacts of the religion, including most of the magnificent monasteries that have existed down through the centuries, but they are incapable of taking the inner spiritual life of the people away from them, as embodied in their systematic use of mantras. A study of the inner life of most Tibetans would still reveal how deeply rooted mantras are in the minds of the people, perhaps especially during the dark hours of these contemporary times. Many Tibetans chant their mantra even while walking, working or travelling. With each step they take, they repeat their mantra in a rhythmical fashion in order to maintain the specific sensation that connects them to their religious practice and in order to recreate the life of spirituality that they know to be at the root of their beings. The repeated mantra creates an uninterrupted mindfulness of the inner vision or recalls it anew into consciousness at will and at any time. The use of the mantra is the key to a higher consciousness, no matter what the external situation or environment conveys. The mantra has the power to connect the practitioner immediately with the various images of the Buddha and the wisdom associated with him. It possesses a magical power that is spiritual at its source, a power that can conjure up a feeling of the immanent reality as well as the knowledge of the one Reality.

The repetition of the sound/word of the mantra and its connections with a higher reality recalls and remembers the Jesus prayer within the Eastern Orthodox tradition of Christianity. St. Paul admonished the Thessalonians to "pray without ceasing," and this is at the heart of the remembrance of the Jesus prayer. The tradition of *hesychasm* was a traditional expression of stillness or repose. The practice of the Jesus Prayer has been well documented in the 19th century classic of Russian Spirituality called *The Way of the Pilgrim*. The pilgrim travels far and wide to learn how to pray without ceasing. He finally meets a *staretz*, a man of advanced spirituality. The prayer "that never stops" is the prayer of Jesus, he is told, a prayer that is formed with the lips, but lies in the heart in order to nurture the inner spirit. It literally brings the person into the presence of Jesus in a manner of speaking, at all times and places, amounting to a kind of Western mantra in terms of its practice and its possibilities. "I grew so accustomed to my prayer," writes the anonymous author of *The Way of the Pilgrim*, "that when I stopped for a single moment I felt, so to speak, as though something were missing, as though I had lost something. The very moment I started the prayer again, it went on easily and joyously."[7]

Whether through mantra, prayer, or sacred formula, the repetition and remembrance of the Immanent Reality through a sacred and revealed vehicle strikes a holy cord within the practitioner that sets in motion a spiritual vibration that leads to a higher consciousness. It amounts to a method that is based on a knowledge that, once internalized, becomes a wisdom that has already proved itself. Method in this sense is actually wisdom in anticipation, while the method itself is simultaneously based on wisdom. It is the interaction of knowledge // action with wisdom // method that actually brings about a marriage of abstract thought with the practicality of an action that has the power to make the abstract real. Through the available method and the subsequent wisdom, the Buddhist monk in search of higher consciousness and the wandering Russian in search of the ceaseless prayer, or the devout Muslim who takes part in the ritual of oral remembrance (*dhikr*), can create and recreate, again and again, a higher reality with the power to infiltrate the seconds, minutes and hours of their days with holy possibility and its

7. *The Way of a Pilgrim*, R.M. French (tr.) (Harper SanFrancisco, 1991), pp. 33–34.

blessed consequences. As part of the traditional setting, these processes represent spiritual disciplines in their most operative mode.

∽

There is no god but Allah. (Quran)

The religion of Islam carries the tradition of the mantra and the Jesus prayer to its logical conclusion with the availability of a sacred formula. Its formal substance in primordial sound and divinely revealed words strikes the holy cord of sacred vibration within the body of the individual and whose inner content of knowledge and wisdom provides in a phrase all that a person need to know in order to get to Heaven. The witnessing, commonly referred to as the testimony of faith, in Arabic the *shahadah*, represents the perfect marriage of wisdom and method, to use the phraseology of the Tibetan Buddhists. Its knowledge reflects the ultimate statement of principle, while its method arises out of the bold affirmation of the truth that is implicit in its repetition and in the actions that are conducted in its spirit. It is the union of wisdom and method, thus representing the meeting of pure wisdom and pure method on the plane of practicality and human experience.

Within the method and wisdom of every act of worship lie both an implicit doctrine and an explicit activity in the form of a spiritual discipline. Prayer, meditation, fasting, pilgrimages, good works, and invocation of the Divine Name are all spiritual forms that convey not only a blessing to the faithful, but also a knowledge and a meaning that can guide them in their daily lives and enhance their spirits. The *shahadah,*[8] which is the quintessential spiritual formula in Islam and the spearhead of a Muslim's faith, does just

8. "This formula consists of two parts: the two first words, which constitute the *nafy* (the 'negation'), and the last two words, which constitute the *ithbat* (the 'affirmation')." F. Schuon, *Dimensions of Islam*, p. 147. Also worth noting is the fact that the *shahadah* is the first sound that the newly born Muslim child hears whispered into the ear, and hopefully the last phrase to part the lips at the moment of death, to accompany the soul on its sacred journey across the divide that separates this world from the next world.

the opposite. It proclaims an explicit doctrine that reflects an implicit activity on the mind and heart of the Muslim believer with its clear knowledge, its active means of discernment, and its dynamic power to move forward, change and ultimately perfect the Muslims in both their inner and external worlds. The *shahadah* proclaims in a phrase that God is the one reality and that Muhammad is His messenger. It is the sacred formula of Islam that summarizes in four words and formalizes in speech the entire substance of the Quran and thus of the religion. In order to resolve the enigmatic mystery that confronts us in the earthly sphere, the Muslim has the benefit of a formal synthesis that is both concise in its expression and rich in its possibilities. The *shahadah* serves this purpose in Islam. For the Muslims, it is a means of spiritual identification, in which they assert what they know to be the essence of a truth that recalls in a phrase the entire substance of the religion.

The *shahadah* summarizes an essential knowledge that draws on the very source of Knowledge itself, and its inward (or outward) recitation becomes the formal vehicle through which to approach and draw near to the Presence of God. It is not only knowledge, it is a sacred emotion; it is not only a theology, it is also a sacred psychology. As the ultimate source of knowledge, the *shahadah* states the truth of the one God and the need for a particular messenger to convey that truth to humanity. If nothing more than the *shahadah* were written in the believer's heart, there would not be need for anything more. As the perfect means of worship and thus of expressing the sacred emotion for God, the testimony of faith that slips off the tongue has the capacity to expand the heart immeasurably. Repeated recitation of the sacred formula brings the Muslim into immediate contact with the truth, physically, emotionally, psychically and spiritually. Through repetition of the formula of the sacred words, faith becomes strengthened until it reaches toward the highest levels of spirituality that are available through the use of the sacred formula. The witnessing is a bold summary of the entire religion, the ultimate motivation, and the absolute foundation of the spiritual life of all Muslims. The Muslim convert becomes Muslim through its official proclamation; the words of the *shahadah* are the first words whispered into the ears of a newly born infant.

Through revelation, God has always proclaimed himself "to exist and be", and has even characterized Himself as the "Hidden Treasure", even if today His existence has been cast into doubt to the extent that people no longer believe in the possibility of a superior Being. Tracing a spiritual line back to one of the earliest religious traditions, we find a similar sacred formula in the Vedantic scriptures in which God also identified Himself as the only reality worth knowing: "Brahman is real, the world is an appearance," thereby establishing once and for all the nature of Reality as well as the true nature of this world as a dream and a mere appearance. Speaking to Moses from the burning bush, God has described Himself in the Bible with these words: "I am that I am" (*Eheyeh asher eheyeh* [Exodus III. 14]). Moses of course did not see the face of God,[9] but he heard God's words, just as humanity has heard the words of revelation down through the millennia, words that have identified God as the Lord and Master of all the creation, including man. Christianity manifests itself clearly through the personality and life of Christ. Nevertheless, it still contains in the Gospels the same essential key with this saying of Jesus in the Gospel: "There is none good but one, that is, God" (*nemo bonus nisi unus Deus*, St. Mark 10:18).[10]

9. If a prophet such as Moses could not see the face of God, then humanity certainly never will. Humans will not see the face of God for the same reasons that they cannot base their faith on seeing the spiritual Reality with their own physical eyes. According to multiple verses of scripture, if such a thing were to happen, humanity would die, or the "mountain would shatter to pieces", thus losing its natural integrity. The Old Testament confirms: When Moses spoke to God, he said: "Show me thy face," and the Lord answered, "Man shall not see Me and live" (Exodus 33:20). The Quran account follows: "When Moses came to the place appointed by Us, and his Lord addressed him, he said: 'Oh my Lord! Show (Thyself) to me, that I may look upon thee.' Allah said: 'By no means canst thou see Me directly): But look upon the mount, if it abide in its place, then shalt thou see Me.' When his Lord manifested His glory on the Mount, He made it as dust. And Moses fell down in a swoon." (7:143).

10. Philosophers, mystics, *walis* and saints down through the ages have passed comment on the nature of the One. It has been a major point of speculation down through religious history in an attempt to reconfirm what has always existed and what lies perennially at the heart of the sacred formula in Islam. Some examples: "There are many numbers, but only One is counted" (Shabistari); "The Self is

The Quran has come not only to proclaim, but also to reconfirm the truth of the one Reality (*al-Haqq*) and the reality of the One (*al-Ahad*). As the final revelation whose messenger seals all prophethood, the Quran makes no pretence of saying something that has never been said before. On the contrary, "for every nation there has been a messenger" (*al-khatim al-anbiya*) that served as the vehicle of the message of truth, and who communicated a universal and perennial truth to satisfy the needs of the people of his time and place. As the final source of the essential knowledge for mankind, the Quran also highlights the identity of the Supreme Being with the phrase "I am Allah, there is no god but I", and the unity of all existence as *the* central doctrine of the entire religion—"He is Allah in the heavens and on the earth" (6:3). As such, the sacred formula of the *shahadah* is a summary statement of all that the religion contains.

⌒

There is no god but I.
There is no god but You.
There is no god but He.
(Quran)

Commentators down through history have made reference to the fact that the Quran is a commentary on the four words of the *shahadah*, and by way of extension, the entire universe verifies and reconfirms the truth of the one reality that is at the heart of all existence. The formula *la ilaha illa 'Llah* is repeated throughout the Quran to remind the faithful of the ultimate Remembrance of God and virtually one third of the Quran is devoted to the knowledge of

---

Brahman, the Self is Vishnu, the Self is Indra, the Self is Shiva; the Self is all this universe. Nothing exists except the Self" (Sri Sankaracharya); "All mankind is in Christ one man, and the unity of Christians is one Man" (St. Augustine); "In God's sight all men are one man, and one man is all men" (Julian of Norwich); "The egg is in the hen, the hen is in the egg: the two in One, and also the One in the two" (Angelus Silesius); "All are really one" (Black Elk); "Therefore the sage keeps to One and becomes the standard for the world" (Tao Te Ching, xxii); and finally, but not the least "For blessedness lieth not in much and many, but in One and oneness" (*Theologia Germanica*, IX).

this explicit remembrance, it being the foundation of the entire religion.[11] In English, it has been translated in various forms including: "There is no god but God"; "there is no truth but the one Truth": "there is no reality but the one Reality". Each of these phrases represents an attempt to express in words the singularity, unity and indivisibility of God in his Essence and all fall short of the profound simplicity of the sacred formula in its original Arabic.

In the Quran, variations of the *shahadah* are expressed alternatively as "there is no god but I"; "There is no god but You"; "There is no god but He". It is interesting to note that the Islamic projection of Allah is not an anthropomorphic God as in the patriarchal, father figure that emerges from the pages of the Bible and the New Testament, nor is the idea of God a fully abstracted projection as is conveyed in Buddhism. Firstly, in addition to the supreme Name of Allah, the Quran identifies ninety-nine names of God and all of them can be used for the purposes of identification and invocation of the Sacred Name. Far from being abstract projections, these names are well-identified and distinctive qualities and attributes that we understand because they are the very qualities that we as humans strive for in order to reflect the higher qualities of the Divine Being. Allah is identified in the Quran as the Nearest Friend (*al-Wali*), the Loving (*al-Wadud*), and the Wise (*al-Hakim*), but these qualities and attributes of character are in fact divine and become human qualities only in so far as our qualities reflect the divine qualities of God. In addition to the divine names and attributes, the use of the divine personal pronouns throughout the Quran lends a personal intimacy and counterpoint to the abstract projection of pure Essence, Being, and Beyond-Being that is otherwise contemplated by esoterics and philosophers.

There is no god but I establishes once and for all the reality of the Supreme Self, alternatively there is no I but the supreme I, in which

11. While the entire Quran is an elaborate and eloquent remembrance of the one God, one third is devoted to emphasizing the truth of the one Reality, one third relates the narrative of sacred history as the model of human behavior to generations of humanity, and one third serves in the form of guidance and advice, threats and warnings, as well as promises to the faithful concerning modes of action in this life and the possibilities implicit in the Hereafter.

the human ego understands the need for the eradication of the individual ego, a purely human and earthly coagulation of psychic and mental forces that must ultimately relinquish its role of indrawn subjectivity in order for the inner self of man to turn instinctively to union with the greater Self of God, the one I, the no I but I. It is the human I vs. the Divine I polarity in which the human being is an appendage and a manifested separateness, the human ego as a microcosm linked with the Divine Self as center and source of the macrocosmic universe. No greater identification is necessary and no greater certainty of a personal, spiritual identity can be made possible for the human entity.

There is no god but You establishes once and for all the special relationship between the human soul and the divine Spirit. "You" expresses none other than the yearning of the self for the Other, Loved One, the Beloved. When man prays, he calls upon "You" with entreaties, supplications and intimacies of heart that need an outlet and voice, partly to escape beyond the confines of the individual self and partly because "You" has virtually become the object of desire, the other-than-the-indrawn self, expressing the deepest yearning of the human soul for fusion with the divine Origin and Source in which the prayerful mind exclaims "there is no you but You." It is the I vs. You polarity in which the human being proclaims the reality of his separateness and the need to reduce that separateness and draw near to the Presence of You, the Other-than-me, the Beloved.

There is no god but He reaffirms the truth that man is not God. He is not I, but rather He is the One who is beyond the individual soul and beyond the individual self as the Other One. He is the third person singular, summoning up feelings of wonder and awe that come with entering the sacred chamber of He. The human being bows, prostrates, prays and praises God because He is the one and only He (*hu*),[12] *la ilaha illa hu, there is no god but He.* Ultimately, man must

---

12. According to the traditions (*ahadith*), the chapter of the Quran entitles *surat al-ikhlass* (112) contains the equivalent of one-third of the Quran in spiritual efficacy and blessing: It reads as follows: "Say: He is Allah, the One and Only; Allah is Eternal and Absolute; He begetteth not, nor is He begotten; and nothing compares to Him."

acknowledge and surrender to the truth that as a human being, he is not He. Only the Divine Being is He and nothing can compare to Him.

The *shahadah* proclaims the existence of Being, the existence of the One, the existence of Existence, remembering the Biblical "I am that I am" and the Quranic "I am Allah". If the *shahadah* were a sacred thread, it would run through all the possible states of existence and penetrate through all dimensions of reality and thereby knit into a unity the very fabric of the universe. If the *shahadah* were a sword it would cut through all ignorance, deception and illusion within man and the world with the knowledge of the one Reality. If the *shahadah* were an icon, it would imprint its sacred image on the mind and heart with its indelible and permanent message of truth. Instead, it is a word that serves as the signature of the Truth. The *shahadah* exposes the myth of the reality of this world and the fiction of the individual self. That man could live and sustain himself without God becomes a tissue of lies, with a texture of unreality that belies man's true intelligence and ability to comprehend both God and the true nature of reality.[13] As such, the *shahadah* is the ultimate thread that connects man to God and the ultimate sword of discernment for humanity who desperately want to know what is real and true. As thread, it weaves the woof and warp of the one reality; as sword it cuts through all ignorance and illusion with the silent blade of Heaven.

∾

This yearning of the mind and heart for an absolute and definitive knowledge is fundamental to the human condition and lies at the very heart the earthly ambition of humanity to transcend themselves and their limitations. This is no truer than at the present time, with contemporary people everywhere still in search of that archetype of the human being represented in the person of the primordial

---

13. "Realizing the first *shahadah* means ... becoming fully conscious that the principle alone is real and that the world, though on its own level it 'exists', 'is not'"; in one sense it therefore means realizing the universal void." Schuon, *Understanding Islam*, p. 17.

Adam and still in search of knowledge of the reality through the pursuit of the knowledge of modern science and technology. Modern and contemporary scientists have come far and achieved much, yet all their accomplishments have a vague air of "unreality" about them because they are missing the one thing essential: namely, the message of the *shahadah*, which is the essential knowledge of the One and the one thing worth knowing when stacked up against all the knowledge of "this world".

Beyond the knowledge contained within the sacred formula, and beyond the discernment between the real and the unreal that is implicit within its message, lies the foundation and key to all spiritual practices. Because the sacred formula of the *shahadah* contains so many spiritual possibilities, because it contains the essential knowledge that virtually summarizes in a phrase the entire religion, because it gives mankind the power to distinguish truth from falsehood, knowledge from ignorance, and the real from the unreal, the *shahadah* contains the seeds not only of an individual practice, but serves as the backdrop and support for all the other spiritual practices of the Islamic spiritual tradition, including the other four earthly duties. "The *shahadah* is not only doctrine, it is also practice—or the key to practice. Its truth is something to be assimilated and lived, which is why, when we speak of the Islamic Credo, we are speaking, not of an abstraction, but of the way in which men and women order their whole lives, their waking and their sleeping, their work and their rest, the words they use in speaking to one another and the gestures they make in loving one another, the planting of a seedling and the reaping of a crop, the turning on of a tap from which water flows and its turning off, and the life and the death of all creatures."[14] The *shahadah*, then, is the fundamental key to all the spiritual practices within the Islamic tradition.

For example, at the center of the prayer ritual lies the knowledge of God as expressed within the *shahadah*, while at the center of the person who bows and makes the prostrations hovers the Divine Presence. The prayer ritual itself is merely the means of bringing the individual soul into the Presence and permitting an intimacy

14. Charles le Gai Eaton, *Islam and the Destiny of Man*, p. 55.

supported by the ritual, together with the words of revelation that soothes hearts and heightens the human consciousness with the remembrance of God. Similarly, the other duties in Islam, the fast, the *zakat* tax on wealth and profit, and finally the *hajj*-pilgrimage have at their center the remembrance of God, which is none other than no god but the one God, for without the meaning and message of the *shahadah* all the other spiritual practices would be superfluous.

The Quran tells us that "man is forgetful"; in fact the grave sin of the Fall from the Paradise is one of forgetting in which Adam forgot God long enough to put himself and his own desires before God. His legacy and the Adamic inheritance, in the Islamic perspective, is therefore to perpetuate within a person's life, thoughts, and actions the act of remembrance of God and the remembrance of the true nature of the one Reality. This is why the emphasis in Islam is on duties or pillars of the religion, spiritual practices that border on the aesthetic and highlight the sacerdotal nature of the human being whose act of remembrance is an individual responsibility of man as celebrant and not by way of proxy through holy intermediaries such as priests or monks. In Islam, every man and women is a priest or nun by virtue of the challenge implicit in the fall from grace and because of the spiritual vocation contained within men and women who have the potential to transcend themselves and therefore their humanity for a higher state of existence.

Unlike prayer, which is required only five times a day, the *shahadah* is the perpetual remembrance. If people could literally transcend their humanity and remain in a perpetual state of remembrance of the existence of the one God and the one Reality, then they would have already recaptured the lost essence of the paradisal man and would have achieved the goal promised to the perfected man. In other words, they would be the primordial man and the perfect man combined in a symbolic merging of eternities. They would once again be one with themselves and they would once again "walk with God". This possibility, however, is not for the average person much less modern individual, who still contains the message of the primordial man and the promise of the perfected man within him or herself as a potentiality and as a fundamental spiritual motive through which to orient their being and their lives. The average man or woman has the other four earthly duties of Islam at their disposal, called the pillars (al-arkan) of the religion, that help them orient themselves toward the remembrance of God and establish a rhythm and a harmony to the days of their lives that are punctuated through the course of time by the remembrance of God.

The Islamic prayer ritual occupies only minutes, but highlights key moments in the rhythm of the day and night, including sunrise, sunset, midday, mid-afternoon, and the moment of total darkness that marks the fifth and final prayer. The fast is the monthly remembrance in which the body itself remembers God through the physical austerity of the fast. The zakat tax on earnings and profit is the yearly remembrance while the Hajj-pilgrimage to Makkah is the once in a lifetime remembrance when the Muslim embarks on a symbolic journey to the very center and hearth of the earth located at the Kaaba in Makkah. In this way, the hours, days, months, years and the very texture of a person's life is shaded and colored with the knowledge behind the face of the sacred formula of the shahadah, even if it is not possible for the average Muslim to maintain the constant second-by-second remembrance that is implied by its perennial repetition of the shahadah and its message of remembrance.

Because the shahadah contains the ternary perspective of knowledge, discernment and spiritual practice, it has all the key elements to form the basis of a sacred psychology of man,[15] a factor which should have considerable appeal to contemporary man who not only needs to find a sound basis to modern psychology, but who also loves to psychoanalyze himself to the extent of "out-psyching" himself.[16] No matter how clever man has become down through the ages

15. "Monotheism is not only a theology; it is also a psychology. As is the Shahadah—la ilaha illa 'Llah." Ibid., p. 59.

16. Surely the modern-day interest in psychology, its very development as a "science", together with the craze of "average man" to pursue the promises of this contemporary psychology, represents the secular answer to the sacred psychologies of the traditions of earlier times, symbolically embodied in the Hellenic phrase "Know thyself" and repeated in variation by the Messenger Muhammad when he said in a well-known hadith: "Know thyself in order to know God."

until the modern times, with astounding developments in technology and science in this last century and with the promises of unlimited developments yet to come, still the human being, on inner levels, is in desperate need to know and understand his own personality, character, and human nature. Even so, we do seem to have sufficient awareness of ourselves to know that the human personality needs to be unified at all levels under a single unifying principle.

We need an image, a center and a straight line that cuts through the fundamental mystery at the heart of the human condition and that gives access to the mystery, focuses our thoughts, and leads us out of and beyond the human predicament. We need an image that provides a model to follow and that summarizes all knowledge at a glance. We need a center that synthesizes the multiple facts and truths that we encounter into a unified and comprehensible whole. We need a straight line that provides the direction and destination to follow as a directive and guiding line of our lives. We need a unifying knowledge that is simple, clear, yet profound, a knowledge who meaning will allow mankind to be well placed within himself, a knowledge that reveals man's true nature as well as the true nature of the reality, and permits him to act out that knowledge in his life. We need to express ourselves as a totality and not as multitudinous fragments scattered across the horizon of our time like broken pieces of glass, shattered by the facility of a world view that separates us further from God and diversifies the inner nature of man rather than unifying man as a clear image, a single line, a center that represents both a reality and a truth. In fact, we need none other than God, who provides the image, the center and the destination that we continue to search for on primary and instinctive levels of our being.

The sacred formula of the *shahadah* contains the summary and synthesis of all that man needs to know in order to express the totality of his being and fulfil his destiny. As such, the Islamic *credo* has been called "the formless form", formless because it embraces and symbolizes in a simple phrase the full range of the entire metacosmic universe and formal because through four simple words—*no god but God*, and three simple ideas—no, yes, and God, it explains definitively and with certainty the inexpressible by identifying for man the Origin, Source, Center and End through the principle of unity and the truth of the one God.

Because the *shahadah* contains the Origin, Source, Center and End within itself, it has therefore the power to bring the believer back to the center of his own being through the power of this centralizing formula. Through the sacred and revealed sound/words themselves, Muslims can establish the vibration, rhythm and melody within their being whose holy cord will reflect back out into the world as a human spirituality most profound. Through knowledge of the doctrine contained within the *shahadah*, they can live out the knowledge of God in life as the fullest expression of their truest self. Through identification with the *shahadah*, the aspiring soul can become simple, clear, profound and transcendent, like the *shahadah* itself. With the sacred formula on his tongue and the Name of God in his heart, he can begin to lift the veil that exists between himself and his own being, and he can cut through the deception, ignorance, and unreality of this world with the sacred formula of the one God.

∾

We began by witnessing the echo of primordial sound as the sounding cord of the created universe, creating physical objects of wonder and beauty through the power of a single cosmic cry. We end with the promise of the celestial rhythms coming down to earth and entering the human soul through the portico of the senses, allowing the soul to participate in the expanding notes of the eternal harmonies. Through sacred sound, human fulfilment in the internalization and realization of God becomes not only a possibility worth pursuing, but a reality worth having.

The lilting voice of the flute over the waters; the delicate whisper of the wind through the trees; the roar of waters through a gorge; the groan of a glacier creeping down the mountainside, the voice of every created thing both animate and inanimate witnesses in their own manner some higher order of magnitude, creating its own rhythm and order of existence and revealing dimensions of reality that would not otherwise be accessible to the human mentality. The phenomena of nature not only exist, they also make themselves known and are true to their nature by becoming audible, visible and subject to smell and taste in order to proclaim some aspect of the essence of what they are. If we listen carefully enough, the hidden message behind the wide variety of sounds that appear in nature poses questions about our true nature and highlight the challenge we face in coming to terms with our own existence, creating waves and vibrations and memory within our inner landscape, what George Elliot referred to as "the unmapped country within us".[17] The wisdom of the senses, once internalized, float across the plain of the soul in undulating waves like the golden wheat in an autumn field ready for harvest.

Imagine for example the sound of snow drifting down out of the night sky like star dust. Its power of silence whispers of some higher dimension that leads toward a deeper and more profound listening, revealing mysteries and insights that previously had been lodged only within the craggy depths of the mind. Once again, it is utter soundlessness that enhances the beauty of sound with its unspoken and sacred absence, recalling the sweetness of Keats' "unheard melodies", arriving one could say at a purity of sound in its very soundlessness, in counterpoint to the cacophony of the world that we have grown accustomed to and that makes us feel alive. If you were the last person on the planet, would there be a need for sound, any more than the need to communicate through words, if there was no one to communicate with? Would the experience of soundlessness complement and enhance the experience of solitude as prelude to the infinite wonder and beatitude that is revealed once the walls of mystery have broken down to reveal the absolute heart of unity and oneness that lies at the center of the universal experience? We do not see the wind, but we know it is there by the visual turmoil of its effect. Arabesques of smoke wind their calligraphic message through the air without a sound. We do not hear the movement of snowflakes but their silent falling on trees and rooftops is more eloquent than any effect their sound could make. We hear the stone splashing in the lake, but the ripples caused by the stone expand endlessly to some distant shore without so much as a whisper. We

17. George Eliot, *Daniel Deronda*, 1976.

see clouds floating through the heavens and observe the shade moving under a tree; but they make no sound except an eloquent silence that hovers upon the threshold of hearing with intensity and dreaminess.

All of the five senses extend their purpose and lend of their wisdom to communicate meaning and reveal the inner essence of an outer physical reality, images through photons of light, sound through rhythm and vibration, scent through its trademark odor and taste through a gustatory experience that brings to fruition the experience of smell. Rather than being perceived as gross and insatiable instruments of pleasure or some crude means of verification of physical reality that we could come to know through touch alone without the beauty and truth of what sight, taste and smell convey, the five senses serve as the arbiters of an unspoken truth, the ultimate mystery that when revealed only leads deeper into the darkness of a universal mystery whose void is reflected symbolically in the image of the universe itself. Objects take on symbolic, indeed metaphysical weight, not only because a crouching spirit lies in waiting behind the physical form, but because we as human beings intuit their significance and choose to believe in their meaning, thus transporting everything into another dimension, into a higher realm of being, into transcendence. What could be just a manifestation of the physical universe becomes something much more because we decide that it should be so. Our spiritual imagination takes us beyond the physical world by anointing and exalting every created thing with the oil of an enduring faith in higher forms of expression. The unknown and unrealized mystery represents a darkness whose silence knocks off the edges of the world and offers some moment of pure, sharp release from our endless wandering in the world of noise, as a flash of lightning freely offers its illumination in the brittle air of a dried-up landscape.

The five senses are candles leading us through the darkness, revealing bottomless shadows that we would never notice on our own. We go through life collecting little insights about ourselves in the world, hoping to preserve a treasured share of light to give away on a special occasion, when we might need a little illumination to resolve a problem or pass through some unexpected misery. Images, smells and sounds create realities that are frozen in time; but that live forever in eternity as celestial archetypes that reflect and recall another plane of existence.

We forget what the forces of nature such as the deserts, mountains and oceans try to remind us of, namely that there is an order of magnitude and levels of existence that extend far beyond anything our own imagination can summon on its own. By speaking of forces far greater than we can possibly invoke and by confronting us with spans of time than we cannot possibly envisage, the experience of the five senses helps us to shape our understanding of ourselves and our place in the universe. The subtleties of sound, as a unique form of communication and as a means of connecting through vibration to the celestial rhythms of the universe, take us out of ourselves every time we hear the song of a bird or the roar of the ocean and lead us beyond our own limited world of forms, opening upon vistas that lie in the mythical land of "beyond", off the edge of the known horizon. Through the resonating power of sound, we are taken to that distant land that shimmers in desert mirages and in sky-high rainbows, or lies beyond the peaks of mountains, where rivers flow and blossoms bloom to a rhythm that transcends sound, awakening us to the reality of the eternal rhythms that float through us like brave clouds across mountain peaks. The sense of hearing raises our consciousness to the point that we can hear the sacred resonance of God in the silent thunder of the Eternal.

5

THE APPRECIATIVE
POWER OF TASTE

Only the one who has tasted knows." (Sufi adage)

Perhaps nothing encaptures more effectively the tempting and transient quality of the sensorial world that we have been reflecting upon within these pages than the sublime sense of taste. As instrument of perception, medium of pleasure and pain, and focus of all that leads us away from the inner side of the reality, our ability to taste the world and all it has to offer promises to drag us down into the depths of the earth to the extent that we are bound by its parameters without the option of ever taking wing and setting ourselves free. The wondrous experience of tasting the world we live in is like the adventure of someone who has to be brought up from the bottom of some deep well. The light is there in the distance as a peephole of promise into the reality of some alternative world; you lie there on your back and are lifted up as though pulling on some internal rope that is none other than the "rope of Allah" sent down to humanity as a blessing and a mercy.

The sense of taste contains a secret that we must discover on our own and a symbolism that resembles an inverted glass, in remembrance of the well known image from the Gospels reminding us that we will experience life as though "through a glass darkly". Before exploring the inner sanctum of the sense of taste and all that it has to offer us in terms of its layered significance, I would like to relate a sober tale in which the much valued sense of taste has been abruptly shut down, at least the first tier of tasting which relates to the pleasurable experience of food and drink as vital nourishment to the body, if not the soul. It is a tale of sad significance, representing a theft of great value, and an incomparable experience of denial and despair that became a force of alchemy and transfiguration in the most unexpected and worthy of souls.

In tribute to the intimate sense of taste, I open this chapter on the miracle of taste by reflecting on the affliction of my older brother who has been robbed of its sublime experience prematurely in life and instead has had to endure an alternative form of tasting in the absolute denial of the taste experience. It is a story in which all of the accustomed pleasure, the sense of appreciation, the communal experience that food inspires, has been abruptly cut out of the broad tapestry of life's experience, leaving the afflicted soul with a loneliness and solitude that cannot be breached from outside or shared from inside. After five years in this condition, my black-belted brother, my mentor, my friend has withered on the vine of life, at least with respect to the physical shell of his body. As for his attitude toward the hand that has been dealt to him and as for the spirit within him, I can only speculate from the signs that he has given me. His spirit shines forth through a body that has given up on him, since he gives very little away concerning his efforts to see his way through this ordeal. The reserves of courage and determination he has had to draw upon cannot be passed on to another as a gift; they can only be witnessed and marveled at from the distance.

His affliction began as a faint tingling in his right cheek over twenty five years ago, a sensation hardly to be noticed, but there all the same, as an uninvited guest into the routine of life's normality. It took twenty years to nurture and grow, but eventually the waif-like numbness and mild tingling became a reality that could no longer be ignored. In the manner of a nightmare that should never come true, the numbness moved with glacial determination down through his jaw, lower face and eventually infiltrated his neck, effectively compromising his ability to control his throat muscles. Suddenly, the dreaded moment had arrived when my brother realized he could no longer eat solid food or even drink liquids. At first, the experience crept up on him on all fours, like the true animal that it was, and he found himself suddenly choking on a small piece of meat and had to be revived with the quick thinking and response to the crisis from one of his sons.

The day finally arrived when the earth stood still and time came to an abrupt halt for him, the moment when the doctors told him, his wife, and sons that he could no longer ingest food or drink. When I first heard the news, I thought of my brother, the broad stride of his gait, his square shoulders and noble head astride a muscular torso, walking into the oblivion of the taste experience, bereft of all the simple, sweet pleasures that we take for granted and would never willingly give up. The blind see inner lights; the deaf hear silence as a profound compensation to the cacophony of the world, the smell of fresh flowers and the subtleties of incense are pleasurable and evocative, but we can live without their unique smells in establishing the cadence and rhythm of our lives, but to lose the experience of taste is to be denied the fundamental plea-sures of the world. The time had finally come when he had to give up all food and drink, forever as they say. For the average person, the word forever has no true meaning; only those who have to face an ultimate denial such as this, the loss of the ability to eat or drink, the loss of a limb, or indeed the loss of a loved one, can understand the true meaning of the word forever in its absolute, final quality.

I had my own taste—for want of a better word—of what the experience of nourishing yourself without actually eating—must have been like for him one winter morning, sitting in the kitchen alone with my brother. When Joseph came into the room and sat himself down for his early morning breakfast ordeal, there was the hint of a smile on his otherwise ravaged face. I felt embarrassed as he stripped off his t-shirt and exposed a frail, pale-white, and shrunken upper torso, as though the very life had been drained out of his body, leaving behind the husk of skin and bone I was now witnessing as testament to his final suffering. The face was actually a visage frozen in endurance and pain, skin and bone covering skull and cranium, giving the appearance that he was a wizened old man far beyond his time. He had difficulty talking; but was a man of few words in any event. I expressed a matter of fact interest in what he was about to do, not knowing precisely what to say; the writer and wordsmith within me feeling much at a loss for words. It was as though time had stood still in this absolute environment. Nothing happened as it should, and yet life flowed on around us, indeed in spite of us. A brilliant winter sun shone through the window. It had been snowing all night in one of those New England winter storms that pass through the area every several years and surprise no one. It continued to drift silently down to the ground in heavy flakes covering the earth in a quilt of white snowy down.

With an abrupt shove, he pushed a sizable tube into the redden opening in his pale white, wrinkled flesh and proceeded to pour down the liquid nourishment that would keep him going for another few hours. Later, he was to wash it all down with a generous portion of clear water, this being the only way he would ingest the pure, life-giving liquid that we take for granted as the vital fluid of the human body. While he nourished himself in this manner and while I sat there with him eating my bran muffin and a plate full of scrambled eggs, unwanted images came to my mind as an equally unwanted silence stood between us, like a thief robbing us of our intimacy. Why did broken eggs shells come to mind, except perhaps for their ragged, dry and fragile quality, for my poor brother looked rather ragged, dried up and fragile as he sat there struggling with the tube while pouring the liquid down into himself. An intense concentration seemed focused on his weathered, aged face. The early morning light streamed in through the Venetian blinds that cast bars of shadow across the kitchen table; but the banners of light drawn across the white table cloth could not outshine or outdistance the determination and dignity pouring forth from the face of my ailing brother.

I didn't know what my brother Joe thought of his ordeal, its reality, its absolute quality, its never-ending aspect, bringing down an endless eternity into the present moment in ways he never expected. He never revealed to me his thoughts. He never spoke about the nature of his suffering, or what he did to overcome his miseries. What we go through life taking for granted, as summarized by the blessed experience of taste, he would never experience again, at least in this life and in this world; yet how did he come to terms with this absolute reality? How did he cope with this perennial misery that he had to face every day of his life?

I secretly suspected that the answer to the question lay somewhere within his brave silence. He never mentioned a word to me about his misery or what it meant to him. During the final stages of his illness, we occasionally corresponded through e-mail. Although the unnamed and undiagnosed disease had continued to spread through his body to the extent that he was put on a portable respirator, he was still able to write lucid letters to me about various items of mutual interest, without ever mentioning his horror, fear, or desperation about the nature of his plight. Out of respect to this silence, I also never mention it. But I am taking the liberty of writing about it now because I think I may have an insight into the true nobility of his character in having passed through this experience in the dignified manner that he has. There is a lesson to be learned here and I am trying to uncover what it might be.

In the same manner that the blind see the shimmering of stars across the field of their dark, inner universe, the deaf hear the music of the spheres and those deprived of the sense of smell take vicarious pleasure in the perfumes of the paradise and the textures available to touch, so also my brother Joseph now lived in a world of higher experience that transcended the lower orders of swallowing caviar on toast and savoring the bubbles of sparkling champagne. If someone had told him in his youth that he would be deprived of his taste buds and would not be able to eat or drink in his later years, he would have dismissed the thought with a wave of the hand as unthinkable. Now he lived in a world that transcended the limitations of the flesh and reached for higher orders of experience on some inner plane of existence, given the complete failure of his outer world and the body that carried him through it. He could have fallen into the dark hole of unthinkable misery, forever longing for that which he could never have again, or worse, succumb to the temptation of falling into a self-pity that would drain the life of the soul in the same way that the vital fluids had been drained from his body.

I believe some invisible door had been made manifest to him that he was allowed to pass through freely, without paying further dues beyond the stark recompense that was already being exacted upon him. Those close to him often marveled in their comments to me that he never mentioned his condition in a negative manner, never complained; indeed never gave voice to the emotive horror that he faced or spoke about it to his loved ones as a means of reaching out for comfort and support. Somehow, he had arrived at a point of detachment and acceptance where no one could follow him, much less understand. He had arrived at some central core whose detachment permitted no sin or pain, amounting to a point of pure experience and a spark of pure truth that allowed him to leave certain aspects of the world behind, a place that belongs solely to God that is not ordinarily at our disposal.

If his body had given up on him, becoming old and decrepit before its time and in defiance to the logic of the normal aging process, so also he seems to have abandoned the myth of the body. In giving up the body's ability to serve his needs, he had transcended its limitations. He was no longer a slave to its needs and demands. Had he then escaped becoming a slave to the reality of his own suffering or did he accept the wings offered to him to fly in defiance beyond the world of the senses? His eloquent silence on the matter seems to answer this rhetorical question.

In coming to terms with his affliction, he had passed through his ordeal to some other side, accepted its reality, and move on into a realm of experience whose inner tasting came from unknown depths, a tasting that only those who have suffered untold loss and survive another day could ever speak of. As I sat in the kitchen opposite my ailing brother that snow-swept morning, a morning whose clear winter light defied the misery of the moment, I began to understand the special gift that he was passing across to me, in his own way and on his own terms. Some wisdom is unspoken, but communicated through example with the power of truth. He had given me a treasure that would enrich me for the rest of my own life, teaching me the meaning of acceptance and endurance, to meet every moment of our lives with the truth that every moment calls forth from us. It is not what we endure, but how we endure it, that captures the essence of who we are.

The Sufi mystic and poet Rumi sings of the human soul as a

symbolic bird in flight: "I am a bird of the heavenly garden. I belong not to the earthly sphere. They have made, for two or three days, a cage of my body." I choose to believe that while the final years of his life were like living in the cage of a body gone wrong, his spirit transcended his misery and was able to fly like a bird. His suffering remained hidden as a form of protection or perhaps protest, withdrawn into the cage of his body with his dignity and spirit intact, like a desert cactus protected by thorns, from the curiosity and pity of the world. Now he has the wings that he has earned on his own terms and has already begun to soar like the eagle flying over rivers and mountain peaks. Whenever I see birds fly across the heavens or a butterfly hovering over a rosebud in search of the taste of life, I will think of my brother Joseph and ask God to grant him the peace that he so richly deserves.[1]

∾

I have embarked on a long, diversionary prelude to these reflections on the appreciative powers of taste because I felt that this was a story that perfectly highlighted the intense, unique, and personal/communal aspect that the gustatory taste experience provides people everyday of their lives and whose absence leaves a chasm as wide as the Grand Canyon. What better way to come to an appreciation of its true value than by recounting the unthinkable possibility of its seemingly absolute denial. The fact is that the sense of taste enriches not only the body, but also the mind, heart and even the soul at all levels of experience and brings people together in ways that would otherwise be unimaginable: the body through the ingestion of food and liquid, the mind as a means of appreciation for the rational and intellectual aspects of life, such as the admiration of a finely exe-

---

1. Not long ago, my brother Joseph passed away, finally giving up the shell of a body that had served him so poorly in his final years. His inner strength and spirit continues to live with those who knew him. I suspect that he would be pleased to know that I have attempted to capture in words the essence of an experience that only he could have understood for sure; but he knew of my love of words and would have appreciated this attempt to describe his experience. In transcending the limitations of the body, he claimed ownership to the wisdom of the senses.

cuted film or the savoring of a well written novel, the heart as an instrument of appreciation of the emotive, the subtle and the beautiful aspects of life that lift us out of ourselves and lead us beyond the threshold of our superficial world onto a high plane of creative spirit well inside the external world of words and forms, and finally the soul as the ground of an experience whose tasting verges on true insight into the intuitive realms that open invisible doors onto the direct perception of the knowledge of God.

Just as the powers of smell derive from an elaborate olfactory network of sense perception that makes it possible at all to appreciate the wide variety of smells at our disposal, so also we can thank our taste buds for their ability to perceive and communicate the broad range of the taste experience from delectably sweet to revoltingly bitter. If we could enlarge our taste buds by viewing them through a microscope, they would look as huge as the volcanoes on Mars. Adults have about 10,000 taste buds in all grouped together according to their specific nature, such as salty, sour, sweet and bitter. Within each group are about fifty taste cells that dutifully relay information to a myriad of neurons that in turn inform the brain of what it needs to know in order to translate sheer form into an experience that we can appreciate. The tongue itself is like a kingdom divided into minor countries according to its sensory talent. We taste sweet things at the tip of the tongue, bitter things at the back, sour things at the sides and salty things all over the tongue's surface. Interestingly enough, they got their name from two 19th century German scientists (Georg Meissner and Rudolf Wagner) who discovered mounds of taste cells that overlap like the petals of a flower. Children have the keenest taste buds of all. A baby's mouth has many more taste buds than an adult. Children love sweets, partly because their tongues are very sensitive to sugar and partly because their taste buds haven't been dulled by years of experience. And like animals, they know what they don't like and will throw to the floor in disgust anything that is not in keeping with their desires.

Taste is first and foremost a gustatory experience of great pleasure through which people nourish their bodies three times a day, not to mention the inevitable daytime snacks and midnight forays to the refrigerator. While the other senses could be called solitary senses because they are essentially appreciated on their own, either through the direct vision of seeing the sublime wonders of nature, the intimate experience of listening to rhythms and the appreciation of the harmonies emitted by every physical thing, or the unique experience of smell that introduces the essence of a thing through the chemical molecules in the air, the art of tasting is usually done in communion with others and therefore could be called the social sense. People generally feel uncomfortable eating by themselves, and dining alone in a restaurant can actually be a painful or embarrassing experience, singling a person out in some unexpected manner since people are not expected to eat alone, much less in a restaurant. We eat with family or friends; business meetings often take place over lunch; weddings always find their culmination in a feast with treasured guests; Irish wakes are notorious for the amounts of food and drink consumed in tribute to the dead, as if in celebration of the life that has now completed itself and passed away. Every culture uses food as a sign of friendship, approval, or commemoration. In Arab and Islamic countries, the celebration of food as a sign and complement to hospitality is a well known aspect of the Islamic culture. I have been invited into Egyptian, Emiratee and Palestinian households and been plied with every manner of food from kusheri, an exotic and layered combination of rice, lentils and pasta, topped off with a thick tomato sauce and sprinkled with pan-fried onions, to stuffed pigeons, considered not only a delicacy in Egypt, but also a special offering to the expectant guest who can savor the succulent pieces of meat as they fall away from the tiny, fragile bones.

At the turn of the millennium and most notably before the iconic date that now defines the ambiance of our time, 9/11, I found myself in a small Pathan village not far from the infamous Khyber Pass in an area that prides itself on hospitality and considers the satisfaction of the guest to be a point of honor as well as the basic etiquette of good manners. We arose early for the ritual prayer before the sunrise, just after the emergence of the first light of dawn, called in Arabic the dawn prayer (*al-salat al-fajr*). Once the prayer was over, we sat down on carpets and cushions strewn across the floor for an elaborate breakfast that included eggs mixed with tomato and spices and fried in olive oil, the famous and oily paratha, to help scoop up the spicy eggs, fresh mango juice served in the form of a milk shake, homemade yoghurt and laban mixed with raw honey, together with a plateful of meat and potatoes swimming in a thick curry sauce. We ate this delectable fare to our heart's content before the hour struck six in the morning.

Several hours later, we were on our way to visit some people in a neighboring village and we were no sooner ensconced in the sitting room next to the inner courtyard, that curiously housed a buffalo, several goats, and a flock of chickens and geese, when we were served an additional spread of fresh fruits and home-made biscuits washed down with white tea, the beloved Lipton fused with generous portions of milk.[2] By ten o'clock that morning, we were led yet again into another inner courtyard that effectively blocked the noise and dust of the village street outside in the public domain. This courtyard was graced by an elegant peacock and a variety of other birds in small wooden cages singing their hearts out, together with the traditional buffalo contentedly chewing on heaps of grass, its dark skin hanging down from its ample torso like an elegant shawl. I was led into one of the inner chambers off the courtyard and was immediately struck by the elegant, leather-bound books all embossed with titles in gold lettering that lined heavy wooden bookshelves along the back and sides of the room. Many of the books were either Qurans or books of *Tafsir*, which are commentaries and ancient manuscripts on the Quran, the sacred traditions or *Hadith* of the Prophet of Islam. Once again, after elaborate ritualized greetings and bear hugs, we sat ourselves down cross-legged on the floor bedecked with beautifully hand-woven tribal carpets. I am always struck when in the company of these tribal people by the ease with which they sit around together in silence without uttering a word, once the ritual pleasantries have been accomplished. One has the impression of calm patience, that there will be time enough to say what one has to say without the inconvenience of being rushed into words that could be inappropriate, misunderstood or offensive. Silence is a luxury these people can afford without being embar-

---

2. Milk is a sign of wealth in Pakistan. If you don't have milk in your tea, it means that you don't have a cow.

rassed by the absence of words; in fact, it is considered a virtue to the extent that one should speak only when one has something of value to say. Silence to them has more value than wasted or empty words.

When in doubt, food is called in, and this was no exception. It was only ten in the morning, but already five hours since the early morning prayer, and this gathering was made historic by my presence: the foreign guest neutralizes all other obligations, social or otherwise. Heaping platters of steaming hot food was soon brought in amid my feeble protests. There were heaping platters of fresh chicken legs and thighs that had been fried a golden brown in buffalo oil, a thick curry of meat and ladies-fingers spiced up with cloves and cardamom, and the traditional chapattis burnished tan, sitting on the platter like folded napkins, steaming hot and invitingly fresh. Amid futile protests, I delicately probed through the spicy curry for a succulent piece of meat and with a finger full of chapatti, I was able to rip off a golden brown wedge of meat from one of the freshly cut chicken thighs whose meat I took note was annoyingly chewy, but delectably juicy, unlike the dried out cardboard supermarket chickens that I had been fed all my life. This too was eventually washed down with steaming cups of hot milky tea.

Having besotted ourselves with food and drink, my friend Farman, the Pathan body guards and I wrapped ourselves up again in our woolen shawls to ward off the winter chill of the morning, made our way back out into the dusty street and climbed back into the waiting jeep. We were on our way to the fish market where we bought several kilos of river fish for the impending lunch. The group of Pathans were very excited about this, and one of them had invited us all back to his house for lunch. After the noontime prayer and having gulped down great drafts of freshly drawn well water from inside the inner courtyard of the house, we all lay supine in a variety of restful attitudes on pillows and cushions strewn across handwoven beds that were set out in the courtyard under the roof terrace to take advantage of the warmth of the noonday winter sun. After much banter and talk among my Pathan friends as they roughhoused with each other in their beloved Pashtu language, fragments of which I was beginning to miraculously pick up: "Sit down, be patient, get out of the way, eat more," was about the extent of my linguistic repertoire, but it inevitably produced gales of laughter and sustained mirth whenever I uttered one of their guttural commands. I also knew how to say the word for meat, and this too sent the other guests into a turmoil of mirth. Younger brothers brought out more piping hot steaming platters of bryiani rice and curry and a variety of Nan breads. Then the fish arrived as if in procession carried across the inner courtyard by a number of younger brothers, several heaping platters of crispy heaping fried fish encrusted with flour and spices.

My oversized Pathan friends, made to seem larger than life by the great encompassing woolen shawls that they sat around wrapped in to ward off the winter chill of the day, dug their great gorilla paws into the rice, meat and fish with expert movements as if they had never eaten before. I was feeling increasingly uncomfortable, unsure whether I would be able to meet the moment and eat a sufficient amount of food to satisfy the strict protocol of the occasion. Hospitality after all is a two edged sword, the host plies the guest with unlimited amounts of food and drink, all delicacies to be sure, and by way of counterpoint, the guest is expected to eat his fill to the satisfaction of the onlookers; anything less than full coverage of all the platters is surely frowned upon. People on either side of me were offering me the choicest morsels of meat and fish. As for the rice bryiani on offer, laden with spices, I had to sift my way through the colorful ménage to make sure that I wouldn't swallow a whole cardamom, a rough edged clove, or a piece of cinnamon bark. I can report that I was at the point of complete distraction and not concentrating properly on what I was eating, when my friend offered me a succulent piece of fish that I swallowed without fully chewing, much less investigating whether there might be an unwanted bone in the midst. Sure enough, I knew that I had problem as soon as I swallowed the bulky ball of rice and fish. A fish bone was stuck in my throat that felt like an old shoe. The story of my journey to a hospital in Peshawar where ultimately the offending bone was assiduously extracted from my aggravated throat has been related elsewhere[3], so I will refrain from going into the details of the mad

3. "Inside Pathan Country", *Sacred Web*, Summer, 2000.

car ride into the city, how my Pathan body-guards ran into the hospital and commandeered the emergency room to protect the "foreign guest" with their trusty Kalashnikovs and my subsequent relief, and the relief of my Pathan friends, when the offending bone was expertly removed by the doctor with a pair of pincers.

By the time we got back to my friend's ancestral home, all the people in the village knew the story of my adventure and were reciting prayers of thanks and gratitude that there was a happy outcome to the tale. This of course called for afternoon tea with biscuits, dried fruits and every manner of nuts and chips spread out across a mat on the sitting room floor, with more visitors coming to welcome me upon my safe return to the village. Plans were already being made for the evening meal, and a great brouhaha was in progress down the garden path and across the street in the inner courtyard of the house of Farman's uncle. He and his family had been planning this event for the entire week, and it was indeed the final night of my visit to the village. A live sheep had been slaughtered for the occasion and it was considered a great honor that this foreign guest would be coming to grace their household. Men from neighboring villages had been invited and were apparently gathering for the great evening repast that was about to take place. I found myself shaking under the folds of my woolen shawl, which I pulled around me now even tighter, partly because of the increasing cold that was creeping across the open courtyard and into the inner sanctum of the darkening rooms of the house where we were gathered, awaiting the signal to move in procession down to the house of Farman's uncle who was waiting with his guests with great anticipation. And indeed I was partly quaking at the thought of having to eat yet another meal on top of the mountains of food that I had already consumed that day, not to mention the unwanted fish bone that was added to the mix.

We all made our ablutions and said the sunset prayer on carpets spread out on the dry mud floor in the courtyard of the ancient house, built like a fortress in this dusty little village. I wasn't sure whether I would be able to eat anything more, and I went through the ritual greetings and salaams of the various guests who shook my hand and embraced me with great warmth and emotion, in addition to their mumbled salaams that is the traditional Islamic greeting.

Many smiles were exchanged, smiles that shone through thick mani-
cured beards, and soon enough the room broke out into the traditional banter that I had come to expect from these social, friendly
people. They were obviously excited by my presence, and my friend
recounted tales to the invited guests of my background, my position
and status at work, my many years as a Muslim, the many countries I
had visited and the many books that I had written on Islam and
other subjects. He embellished his tales with great exaggeration and
verve, much to the delight of the onlookers who nodded approv-
ingly and rested their smoky eyes on me with warmth and blessing. I
could see their cold breath emerge as icy smoke into the frigid night
air as I sat there myself chilled to the bone.

I sat there cross-legged and propped up on cushions, looking
demure and exuding an air of agreeability, as though through a hint
of a smile and a twinkle of an eye, I were attesting to the veracity of
the tales my friend was recounting. Needless to say, I didn't feel the
slightest bit hungry and longed for the days of fasting when the
Muslims go the entire day without food or drink until the call to
prayer at the sunset. I was beginning to realize, in spite of my honored status as beloved foreign guest, the joys of hunger up against
the miseries of fullness and satiation that comes with overeating.
The Quran informs us: "Eat and drink, but do not be extravagant."
(7:31) Never again would I long for black forest cake or baked ziti. I
had had my fill of food to last me a lifetime. Still, it wasn't long
before a plastic floor cloth was laid down across the sitting room
carpet and heaping platters of hot food was spread across the floor.
Secretly, I vowed never to eat again and promised myself to take up
fasting as a permanent ritual, affording a deeper pleasure than any
culinary dish could ever offer me again. Somehow, I got through
the evening of celebration to the great hospitality of these Pathan
people, who honor their guest in many ways, not the least of which
by plying the unsuspecting guest with platters of food to their
heart's . . . content.

It is a humbling experience to be fully accepted and taken into the
inner circle of a family and the warm embrace of village life, indeed
into an ancient and traditional tribe who practice very conservative
customs and follow strong religious beliefs. The Pathan people

seemed to me larger than life, physically, mentally, and spiritually. Physically, the appearance of many of them was that of the lovable giants of legends and folk tales. You come to know them, however, through their actions and not their words, for the extent of their generosity knows no bounds and the needs and comfort of the guest takes precedence in all matters. The face you see is their true face. The words you hear are their true words. If they take you in, you are one with them. They showed an attitude toward me that made it clear they considered me their brother and friend. It was unexpressed in words, but spontaneous and freely offered through their actions and behavior. No matter who I was or where I had come from, to them I was now Pathan and one with them. This was no journey of a stranger in a strange land. On the contrary, this was a journey in which my soul felt at home. If I were asked where I was and how I got there and why, I could have given a clear answer because I had found one in the encounter with these simple tribesmen.

On a number of occasions, I was asked, perhaps a little self-consciously, what I thought of the Pathan people. It was a question I was instinctively reluctant to answer, partly because I felt that no simple answer existed or came to mind that could do justice to the experience I was having, and partly because it would take serious consideration and the right words to portray the greatness and nobility of these people in their true light and could not be summarized in a few superficial words. In writing this tribute, I have finally answered this question as I promised I would, a promise that needed to be kept in view of the profound outpouring of sentiment this great tribe had extended toward me.

❧

"Oh those who believe! Fasting is prescribed to you as it was prescribed to those before you so that you may learn heedfulness." (Quran 2, The Cow, 183)

In counterpoint to fine culinary dining and the savoring of exotic drinks from fresh fruit juices to the finest wines, the Islamic traditions turn the sense of taste inside out through the Islamic fast, based on the premise that hunger rather than satiation of the senses will turn the mind away from the temptations of the sensible world to the inner world of higher experience, when the eye of the heart and the intellect opens wide and the sheer experience of formal denial of the taste experience, at least for a temporary and limited time frame, will open a door to the conscious experience of a higher order. When the physical eye sees the sun, moon and stars, the inner eye witnesses the singular reality of the Creator who created the formal universe and set humanity at its very center to witness and surrender. When the Muslims set out to systematically deny the pleasures of the sense of taste, they put their surrender into an action that is the direct expression of their will to surrender to the commands of Allah.

Muslims the world over fast during the lunar month of Ramadhan first and foremost because Allah has asked them to do so in the verses of the Quran. When the Divinity asks, the true Muslim complies. If this were the only reason why they fast, it would be reason enough. Muslims believe the Quran to be the direct communication of the Divine Being to mankind, a revelation that provides the essential knowledge they need to know in order to realize their spirituality as a living spirituality within the context of their lives. It is not, however, the only reason. The Islamic fast has a spiritual significance and efficacy that ranges from purely external benefits to profoundly internal blessings. Embedded within the ritual of fasting, however, there lies a spiritual meaning, a human secret, and a divine promise that forms the rationale and purpose of the entire body experience of the fast.

In its external manifestation, the fast of Ramadhan is a well known phenomenon. Most people know that fasting calls to a halt the satisfaction of the appreciative sense of taste for a specific time period from the call to prayer at the first light of dawn until the call to prayer at sunset. The rhythm of normal life is sharply interrupted, while the Muslims adapt themselves to the routine of self denial implicit in the fast. The fast is an intense physical effort in which the body experiences a kind of death to the satisfaction of the senses, in keeping with the traditional saying (*hadith*) of the Prophet: "Die before you die."

The fast of Ramadhan is a form of worship in which the body

itself offers up its own prayer as it passes through a netherworld that denies all sense experience relating to taste. Because of its message of effort and self discipline, the fast is a most effective way of conquering the evil within us. The Prophet of Islam has said: "Satan affects the sons of Adam by pervading his blood. Let him therefore make this difficult for Satan by means of hunger." The fast denies the senses their natural satisfaction because they are the "grazing ground" of the devil. As long as the senses are fertile, the devil will continue to frequent them and as long as he frequents them, the majesty of God will not be revealed to the human consciousness.? "Had it not been for the fast," the Prophet said, "the devils would hover around the heart of the children of Adam, when in truth the fast would have lifted their hearts unto the kingdom of Heaven." For this reason, the Prophet also told his favorite wife, Aisha, "Persist in knocking on the door of Paradise." When she asked how, the Prophet replied: "With hunger."

The physical efficacy of the fast has been well documented down through history, and most religious traditions have encouraged fasting. Even the secular societies of the West recognize the benefits of the fast and have included fasting as an important factor in the pursuit of good nutrition and health. In fact, fasting has been called "the bread of the prophets" because it is virtually a prayer of the body. Fasting helps the body to purify itself of the toxins that accumulate through over-indulgence of good foods and incomplete digestion. The resulting purification leaves the body in a more refined state of physical readiness and awareness. Through denial, the physical senses are actually heightened; some of the veils that separate us from the higher realities may be lifted, and the remembrance (*dikhr*) of Allah is brought clearer into focus. The body itself goes through a process of fine tuning, so that a person can begin to listen to the message that the body has to convey. As Rumi, a well known Islamic mystic from the 13th century wrote in one of his poems: "If the brain and belly are burned clean with fasting, every moment a new song comes out of the fire."

Beyond the boundaries of the external fast lies the internal fast. Internal fasting imposes a discipline on the mind and soul. The inner self is restrained from indulging in passions and desires that go beyond the physical senses to affect one's personality and inner psyche. These are the inner evils such as lying, backbiting, envy, jealousy, anger or pride. "Cultivate within yourself," the Prophet said, "the attributes of Allah." The internal fast transcends the physical limitations of an individual and amounts to imitating the qualities of God. With its inward focus, the fast weakens the knots of the psyche, controls the negative emotions of the personality, and strengthens the human will that initiates the fast in the first place. In this way, the human spirit becomes stronger both outwardly through control over the senses and inwardly by focusing the mind and transcending the limitations of the psyche. Those who do not fulfill the minimum conditions of both the outer and inner fast are the people about whom the Prophet has said, "There are many whose fasting is nothing beyond being hungry and thirsty."

Of all the earthly duties, the fast of Ramadhan is the most secret because it is strictly between the individual and God. The fast by its very nature is an act of honor and a secret pledge between man and God. The prayer rituals, the *zakat* payment and the Hajj pilgrimage are all open to plain view and subject to comment and approval by the community, whereas the fast is the one act of worship that is witnessed only by God. People who fast cannot prove their veracity and don't have to; rather they share their secret with no one but the only One, in obedience to God and for His sake only.

All five pillars of Islam have the remembrance of Allah as their fundamental motive and purpose. This is obvious in the first duty, the proclamation of faith (*shahadah*), which is the perpetual remembrance of the one God and the one Reality. According to the Prophet, the prayer is the "key to Paradise". By observing the *zakat* or giving of alms, the Muslims remember Allah through their earnings. The pilgrimage brings us back physically as well as spiritually to the center of the world, the Ka'aba in Makka, which is also the symbol of the inward center, the heart, which is the place where the remembrance of God becomes a meeting ground and a reality. Finally, the main purpose of the fast is the achievement of a state of detachment from the world through the outright denial of the senses, in order to create a space within the mind and heart for the "remembrance" (*dhikr*) of Allah. This is perhaps the greatest and most immediate benefit of the fast, for Allah has said: "Remember Me and I will remember you" (2:152).

The fast of Ramadhan ultimately contains a meaning, a blessing, and a promise that extends far beyond human expectations or experience. "Fasting is for Me and I shall grant reward for it Myself." In compensation for the human effort of the fast, the divine promise has both an outer and an inner aspect. The two joys of fasting are the *Iftar* or "break-fast" meal that concludes the fast and the vision of the new moon that signals the *Eid* at the termination of Ramadhan. The inner blessing is what modern psychological terminology would call a higher consciousness or "presence of mind" together with a feeling of serenity and peace that accompanies any strong effort of human will, in this case a virtual surrender to the Will of God. In Quranic terminology, this is called *tatma'inn al-qulub*, a peace that descends on the hearts of the believers from above as a foretaste of the ultimate divine promise, namely the joy of seeing the paradise (*jannah*) after death and the beneficence of having the vision of God after resurrection.

∽

Is it any wonder that the sense of taste ties us initially and inevitably to the sensible world that we enjoy and relate to through all of the five senses? Because taste binds us to sustaining life through ingestion and nourishment, and because its first tier significance links us to the pleasures it has on offer, we may well become negligent and fall prey to the temptation of overlooking, if not actually ignoring, the inner aspect of "taste", or what the Sufis in the Islamic tradition call *dhawq*. If we have learned nothing else from our study of the five senses and our reflections on their possible input into the realization of a higher order of experience, we have finally come to realize that the senses and the mind[4] cannot be fully relied upon, if we

---

4. In that regard, the human senses play a similar role that the various human faculties, such as the faculty of reason, human intelligence, the higher sentiments and emotions, not to mention the heart knowledge that lies at the center of our being.

remain only within the first tier of their experience, without looking beyond their superficial import to the deeper experience they have on offer.

In the Islamic worldview, the body exists as a vehicle within the world of the *dunia* (this world) and as a conduit and reflection for the tendencies of the soul. The body is conceived as a kingdom; but the soul is the king, while the intellectual faculties and human senses are the cohort and army in coming to terms with reality within this vast, microcosmic world. Beyond taste as nourishment lies taste as appreciation on the physical, mental and psychic planes of experience. In the traditional Islamic view, the human mind has the capacity to ingest and appreciate—to taste if you will—intelligible, intelligent and intellectual input that comes to us from the outside world in the form of the arts and crafts and the good works that others have accomplished. To read and appreciate a great piece of literature, to bask in the vision of a work of sacred art, to absorb the visual artistry and experience the profound meaning in the utility of a well-wrought handcraft such as a traditional carpet or a hand-carved brass serving tray is to absorb the creative, intellectual and higher level spiritual experience of another person into oneself as a means of enlightenment, such as the appreciative tasting of a book, the beauty of a sacred work of architecture or a handwritten parchment of calligraphy.

No one wants to be tied forever to the sensible world. It is not the world as such that draws a deep attraction out of us; but rather its beauty, utility and the love it generates that inspires our deepest emotions. Even if people are attached to the world, they eventually are given the wake up call of death that cuts short the sense experience as we know it in this world. The challenge of the senses is to use these five windows to the world to piece together the fabric of the sensible reality with the wrap and weft of a higher perception. The religious traditions tell us that the metacosmic reality is the ultimate reality and that the five physical senses play a vital role in leading humanity to the knowledge of a higher reality and the experience of a supra-sensible spirituality that is not bound by the physical and sensible world. The experience of the senses contains the elements of a reality insofar as, through their enjoyment, they provide an inkling of a higher purposeful reality or through their denial and the implicit inner purification and heightened consciousness implied by such a denial, they lead us beyond the sheer experience of the physical world. The five senses that we rely on so heavily to negotiate our way through this world become the stuff of pure illusion when they express an independence from the source of their true reality, or worse, are used as instruments in the identification and verification of some reality they proclaim to be true "on their own"!

The secret of the senses lies in their ability to transcend their own limitations and their first tier significance as portals of pleasure and nourishment on the purely physical plane for an experience of the mystery of the Divinity that the Gospels refer to, when Jesus said: "Eye hath not seen nor ear heard, nor hath it entered into the heart of man.[5] The mind is normally so distracted by the senses from its true mission to rise above itself and perceive the higher realities, that it needs first of all to gain some mastery over the demands of the senses and become withdrawn from the complete domination of external things over the inner psyche of humanity. Do we ever think of God when we taste a date or a fig? Do we ever remember our Lord and Master when we see a rainbow or lightning streaking through the sky like a flaming sword from Heaven? The unique essence of taste, as in the unique essence in the smell of a lily, finds its original source in its unique archetype on the other side of reality. Their taste conveys a universal quality that touches every heart as well as every taste bud with its irresistible mystery as well as its unqualified magic, proclaiming "we did not make ourselves; but He who endureth forever has made us."

We know that the senses—and especially the sense of taste— convey a knowledge of sorts, but how we appreciate that knowledge and absorb its inner content will ultimately reflect upon the kind of person we are and the kind of person we will become through the manner in which we ingest and appreciate the wisdom of the senses. Are we as individuals suppose to follow the guidance of the modern, secular worldview that has tied up human reason and the experience of the five senses into an exploratory pursuit of knowledge

5. 1 Cor. 2:9.

whose point of departure is the physical world and whose ulti-mately destination—such as it is—lies presumably within the innu-merable and infinitely miniscule particles that are found at the quantum physical level of experience, at the expense of the world of first principles and universal knowledge that lies at the heart of the traditional, metaphysical worldview. It recalls the efforts of the spi-der, who not only spins its own web with the materials that has been providentially laid at hand; but who climbs up and down and across its own little universe, pinned to the experience of its own reality in the same manner and perhaps in just compensation to the way in which it traps its prey for its own purposes.

What begins as a first tier experience that involves the tasting and appreciation of the physical world has the power to become a soul experience with far-reaching proportions. What begins as a tasting and an appreciation on the bodily, mental and psychic planes of experience eventually comes to rest within the ground of the human soul as an inner awakening to a higher experience of consciousness. Within the Islamic context, it is not a given that the soul partakes of an innate spirituality; rather the soul represents the summary and culmination of the human experience across a broad spectrum of good and evil inclinations, leading the soul to become a mirror reflection of all that we know and do in this life, either as victim to the insatiable senses of the senses or as benefactor to what the senses may reveal. The soul is the expression of who we are. The Turkish poet Yunus Emre has summarized the concept nicely by putting his finger on the pulse of the true significance of the sense of taste and how that relates within the deep well of the soul experience:

> When I eat something sweet without You, it's bitter.
> You are the soul's taste, what else could I want? [6]

It has been said that when the hungry man sees the sight of steaming hot bread, his instinctive desire is equal to the aspiration of a thousand seekers of truth. We need to feed off our hunger as an alternative experience of taste with the power to transform our soul

6. As quoted in *Music of the Sky*, 'The Drop that Became the Sea', p. 73, "Music of the Sky".

into a mirror reflection of the Divinity. The Sufis of the Islamic tradition refer directly to *dhawq* as an experience of taste that relates to
the experience of spiritual intuition that is the immediate result of
the direct perception of the faculty of the intellect of the knowledge
of God. Only the direct experience of the knowledge of God as the
ultimate experience of taste can bring to fruition the entire range of
human yearning to transcend the physical plane of experience. Ibn
'Arabi told a disciple: "If someone enjoins you to prove the existence
of the 'knowledge of divine secrets', demand that they in turn prove
the smoothness of honey." I think what Ibn 'Arabi was referring to
was not the superficial experience of taste that comes from the nectar of honey or the sweetness of the fig. The experience of higher
spiritual consciousness and its corresponding path of awakening
begins with the gustatory knowledge of the world, with the smoothness of honey and the tart quality of the lemon, the sweetness of
fresh dates and the soothing quality of mother's milk, partly
because they give what they have to offer without exacting an undue
price and partly because they have retained the taste of the paradise
that is their inborn nature.

Perhaps we should invoke the words of Al-Hallaj, a well-known
Sufi who was put to death by crucifixion because of his unorthodox
proclamations, to help us remember the inner meaning of the taste
experience, when he proclaimed: "When I wanted to drink to
quench my thirst, it is You that I saw in the shadow of the goblet."[7]
Let us give thanks at the table of life for the provision (*rizq*) that has
been bestowed upon us and appreciate it as the sweet blessing that it
is intended to be. Let us lift up our cup and bowl in salute to the
provision that has been sent down to us from the Supreme Provider
"for many a slender beauty heaven has made into a hundred cups, a
hundred bowls.[8]

7. *Return to the Essential* (Bloomington, IN: World Wisdom Books, 2004), p. 5.

8. Omar Khayyam, *Music of the Sky* (Bloomington, IN: World Wisdom Books, 2004), p. 120.

6

THE EXPLORATORY
POWER OF TOUCH

And I have felt
A presence that disturbs me with the joy
Of elevated thoughts; a sense sublime
Of something far more deeply interfused,
Whose dwelling is the light of setting suns,
And the round ocean and the living air,
And the blue sky, and in the mind of man.
(from Tintern Abbey, William Wordsworth)

After reflecting upon the hidden spirit and wisdom of the other four senses, arriving at the fifth and final sense of touch is a little like opening the bottom draw of a bedroom dresser hoping to find that which you might have lost was merely tucked away for safe keeping, a secret treasure waiting once again to see the light of some eternal day. We hope to uncover one final instrument of perception that will serve our needs in identifying the true nature of the physical world and help us negotiate our way through its labyrinthine passageways, like blind men in a forest of trees, hoping to arrive at an illuminated knowledge that will bring us to the moment when the light of the senses is extinguished by a flash of lightning that has revealed the invisible world by making it visible.

In coming to terms with the full extent of the sense of touch and what its offers us in terms of knowledge of the world and insight into ourselves and others, we may find that we have uncovered a very special treasure indeed. By robbing the intrinsic value of the sense of touch as a means of objectifying the physical reality, we may find much more wisdom embedded within the sense of touch than we ever bargained for on the purely physical plane of existence. The price of this wisdom may force us to leave behind the treasured illusion that the physical senses have the power to substantiate the reality on their own, without the aid of Heaven.

Touch is a unique sense that seems to have no fixed abode, inclining me to suggest that it is the subtle sense. Touch is not embedded within our head like the ears, eyes, nose and mouth of the other senses and we tend to forget about its impact on our lives until we reach out and touch someone or are touched in return. As the delicate and non-specific sense on many levels, touch is unlike vision and its complement the eye, the characteristic nose that adorns the central portion of the face; the floppy ears with passage-ways that reach deep into the brain with their revelatory sounds or the tongue with its hills and valleys of taste buds with the power to rock our satisfactions with joy. We have suggested that the eye is not some little orb, closed off from the visions of the miraculous in a darkened world of colored shadows, nor the ear a little shell of small volutions shutting out the true echoes of celestial sounds from the harmonies of the natural order, nor the nose as some fleshy viaduct to facilitate a neutral and odor free air into the cor-poreal system as oxygenated blood and enlivened cells. Each of the other four senses have their own private research center and instru-ments of investigation with which to explore the physical and natu-ral order with a view to revealing its hidden mysteries. Touch, on the other hand, has the skin of the body as its primary organ and the human hand as its instrument of exploration, although in truth, almost any part of the body is technically capable of making discreet inquiries of their own, thus making the body its own elabo-rate sensory system.

It is as if we climb into our bodies at birth to take up habitation in the world, or put on our bodies like a cloak of many colors with aspects that protect us from the elements; yet all the while actually having the power to prevent us from escaping the limitations of the physical world that we continually bump up against through the medium of the five senses, whereas the true goal is to escape the car-nal world of the senses and the prosaic world of touch in order to set about the task of perceiving God's presence in the world. The skin that harbors the sense of touch envelopes a body that itself becomes the instrument of sensorial exploration, as well as the vehicle of sensuous wonder and delight. In a sense, we can envision it as though climbing into a tailored suit or putting on a kit glove, or perhaps we should envision the instrumentation of touch as the pure white envelope into which the soul has been placed in order to make its unique journey through life in search of an absolute that transcends relative polarities of this world.

Inside the envelope of the skin, something sacred dwells. The sense of touch and the skin that is its receptacle is all about surfaces and sensation; but on deeper levels and as object of desire for the sense of touch, the skin is to the soul what a map is to a landscape, a useful reduction of reality whose markings and signposts can lead us back with its implicit guidance to the true inner reality that we are reaching out for. In a sense we can claim that touch is the oldest sense and perhaps the most urgent. No other sense can affect people like the sense of touch and as such could be call the prime vehicle of the emotions. Our bodies are what carry us through the world, but our skin and the sense of touch that it relies on is all that stands between us and the world. The skin itself is alive, a living, breathing and indeed excreting shield, protecting us from the harmful rays of the sun and microbial attack of bacteria and germs, insulating us from heat and cold and repairing itself when necessary. As the largest organ of the body, the skin weighs from six to ten pounds and serves as the key organ of sexual attraction. It makes up about 16 percent of our body weight and stretches two square yards.

It takes our entire infancy and well into childhood to become accustomed to the house that we must inhabit and much of this acclimatization of the body with the world comes about through the exploratory powers of touch, getting to know and experience the texture and feel of the world around us. Infant babies first use the sense of touch before all the other senses to explore the world around them. There is an instinctive knowledge in touch the allows the demanding infant to find the mother's breast whence taste clicks in through the sucking motions of the mouth and tongue in ingesting the comfort and nutrition of mother's milk. It is as if infant babies begin life as human sense machines and in all frankness enjoy all of the ambiguous wonder of the physical world. The poet Thomas Traherne speaks on behalf of the infant child when he marvels: "How wise was I in fancy! I then saw in the clearest Light." He celebrated "sweet infancy" as another world, a different universe, in which "the first impressions are immortal all."[1] In exploring its world initially through the sense of touch and soon followed by the other senses, the infant moves through a garden of childish delights where every cloud is a dragon and every bird chirps its sweet song of enchantment as it floats through the wind. My little grandchild Raouf may shed childish tears of sorrow at some slight or unhappiness, but I needed only to pick him up into my arms and point to the trees, imitating the tweet-tweet of the birds, to transport him out of his misery as if by touch into his inner world of magical enchantment. Like dew falling from a leaf, his tears fall from his face as it breaks open with laughter. Without the encumbrances of the mind and the complexes of the adult psyche, the child plies through its world as an artist and visionary, exploring through touch, taste and the other senses the magical wonders of what seems like some primitive, paradisal world. Thoughts, dreams and inspirations come to us later as compensation for the loss of infant fantasy, but nothing can compare to the raw, spontaneous and virgin nature of the infant's exploration of its immediate world, making them all explorers and visionaries.

On the subject of the princely state of infancy, when images of fire-flies and faeries float freely through their uncorrupted minds like butterflies in search of nectar, when the waking state actually resembles a dream come true in that everything is still fresh, distinctive and pure, and when the imagination roams freely through the images of the world and become what a child imagines them to be without any cloud or encumbrance, I recall an intimate moment of encounter with my two year old grandchild that I shall never forget, a moment that seemed as if God Himself had reached down into the infant child's tender little heart to reach out and touch me

1. Theodore Roszak, *Where the Wasteland Ends* (Garden City, NY: Doubleday & Co., 1972), p. 326.

with His compassion and love through the medium of the child. That is what struck me at the time and that is what I remember. The baby Raouf has already moved on to another time; the moment has passed and he will change and grow to be a man, but to me he will always be a reflection of God reaching down to touch my heart with the love of an infant child and to whisper of His mysteries through this poignant human encounter.

I had journeyed up into the northern-most reaches of the North West Frontier of Pakistan to visit a Pathan family that I had grown very close to while working in the Middle East. My Pathan friend Farman and his wife had six children who had grown up thinking that I was their grandfather, which only attests to the simplicity and the child-like quality of acceptance and love that young children freely extend to those who love them in return. Although I came from another world halfway around the globe and did not look like the rest of their extended family and tribe from their village, these young children behaved as though I were one of their own. Each of the children vied with one another to claim that I was "their" Baba and no other elder in the village could claim that right.

The village itself was in various stages of shutting down for the night as we approached it in the winter fog. It was dark enough as we made our way through the one dirt road full of cracks and holes and framed on each side with the crumbling mud walls of the houses and shops of the village. The lights had apparently gone out and inside the shops I could see the flickering of candles. People were making their way through the darkness on foot or on motor-cycles slicing through the darkness with their headlights and noisy clatter, but everyone deferred to the movement and progress of the car. Suddenly, we had arrived and I was unceremoniously shoved down the dusty path and around the corner between stately poplar trees. I heard the chatter and singing of children and then saw them standing in a cluster in silhouette against a hanging lamp in front of the door of the house where they lived. When they saw me, they came running forward in a cascade of glee, sounding like birds in a tree at sunset. Shouting Baba, Baba in their unrestrained excite-ment, they threw flower petals over my head and shoulders as tears came to my eyes. Then each of them salaamed me respectfully and extended their little fingers for the traditional handshake. I noticed through the hubbub that they were scrubbed clean and neatly dressed, the girls' heads wrapped discreetly in the colorful Pathan shawls. My arrival was an occasion that they had anticipated and prepared for the entire week.

Raouf, the baby now one and a half years old, sat contentedly in the arms of Farman's oldest brother, Niaz Mohamed, who himself stood next to the children looking like the Grand Mufti of Al-Azhar, the famed Islamic university in Cairo, with his majestic face and sculptured white beard. Raouf sat there as if he owned this niche and had every right to be there, his little legs dangling barefooted from the shelf of Niaz's strong arm in careless abandon. Niaz Mohamed walked over through the darkness of the night and immediately handed the baby over to me. It has been three months since Raouf sat contentedly in my arms. Once there, he could have stayed there for all eternity to the extent that whenever I wanted to put him down, he protested mightily. However, some time had passed and at that age, I wondered whether Raouf would remember his Baba. Would the adorable baby Raouf remember this aging bag of bones that he had once clung to and cherished as his beloved Baba.

I had been told by Farmana that in order to perpetuate my memory, they would show Raouf my photograph and he would proceed to march around the house showing everyone and pointing to his Baba, the first and only word that he could yet articulate, uttering the sound like some secret, lost revelation newly discovered. In my mind as I had prepared for the trip and now as I stood there at the true moment of my arrival, I wondered if he would remember me. I had lived a long and interesting life and accomplished many different things; but the recognition of the baby Raouf and his sweet remembrance had suddenly taken on vital importance to me, the only moment worth waiting for and that needed to come true. Worlds could turn on their orbit and eternities pass us by, but if this beloved infant didn't remember me, it would lay waste my new world and shatter the fragile expectation we having of loving and being loved in return. There is something primordial and unique in the outpouring love of an infant baby. There are no conditions or self-conscious attachments associated with this raw emotion; it emerges from the noble presence of the child with its own spontaneous, primitive and unconditioned truth. It seems to ask nothing in return and in so doing opens a world of love and emotion that pour out willingly from soul to soul like flood water spilling over a dam. Infants recognize true love in others and give it back freely in return; otherwise they may not have anything to do with you.

Judging from the size of his eyes and the hint of his smile, Raouf was clearly caught up in the excitement of the moment as he was passed into my arms before he had time to think about it or protest. As he settled his chubby frame into the crook of my arm where he had spent so many weekends during what seemed now like the ancient history of our time, he wasn't sure he was having any of this, momentarily confused by the excitement of the moment and the shouts of the other children. I could see in his eyes and attitude that he wasn't sure who I was at first and was going to take his time making up his mind. He sat there in my arms eye to eye and face to face and began to scrutinize precisely the true person he was seeing before him. I have always marveled at the child's ability to being fully in the moment without the contrived context and excess baggage that adults usually carry around with them, and this moment was no exception. Raouf took me in with all the instinctive powers available to him as an infant presence, like some regal prince surveying one of his subjects. At first he seemed to roam the topography of my face for some familiar landmarks and for a second he raised his pudgy little fist and touched my beard, as though feeling its texture for hints of the identity of this strange person causing so much excitement; then not getting a satisfying reply from this brief survey of touch, I saw the child look straight into my eyes and I stared back, his head seemingly surrounded by a halo in a mist of light.

This was no casual glance; I could feel him probing deeply into the well of my being for a signal that would awaken his memories, as though he were searching through the forest for a glimpse at a passing deer or scanning the horizon of a great ocean for signs of land. For a moment, his gaze was so penetrating and direct, I felt as if I were suspended in mid-air without any ground under my feet, held aloft by the scrutiny of his pure, uncluttered gaze; my heart had become merely a string that was being pulled taut so that I could actually feel pain. Then, without further ado, this boy wonder made up his mind, gave me the most beatific smile imaginable and uttered distinctly the word Baba, as though he were intoning notes from a piece of musical script and Baba again and again, setting up echoes in my heart of a distant bell whose reverberation ran through my being like the sounding notes of some grand adagio, and I was thinking that we had just journeyed together to the world's edge and had come back with smiles on our faces. It filled my heart with joy to know that the traditional loyalty and faithfulness was already there in the little heart of this Pathan infant. We all made our way into the house together; but my eyes were glistening and wet as I carried this contented little mountain man in my arms through the front door.

I recall the sweet memory of this episode in which age and infancy come together through some unspoken communal bond because it highlights to perfection the two-edged sword that characterizes the true sense of touch. It is a narrative that reaches beyond the superficial benefits of touch toward some deeper sensory participation in which two individuals touch each other not with their fingers or hands and not even with their minds, but solely with the sentiments of the heart, the interaction of a heart-emotion that transcends the physical, sensorial plane of bodily touch in order to manifest an intuitive power within each of the senses, and most notably in the sense of touch, when we touch the heart of another and are touched in return. There is a ghostly quality to touch that transcends the grainy quality that comes with merely touching the surface of things. The encounter with the baby Raouf had a physical correspondence comparable to touching silk or velvet cloth and recalls the smoothness of honey on the tongue. If you can explain the true nature of the experience or define its quality in words that go beyond the physical interaction, or if our sensorial impressions pass through doors of perception that have been cleansed or are the expression of a purity of heart that only an infant child can summon, then everything would appear to us as it is in truth, as the expression of the Infinite.

◠

Trust to what the senses show.
There's nothing false in what they know.
(Goethe, *Vermächtnis*)

I would be remiss in my duty and in the dictates of common sense if I did not mention within these pages the word sex in dealing with the sense of touch. In the physical contact of one body to another, there are powerful sympathies working their way deep into the flesh for their satisfaction, just as the other bodily senses find in things certain qualities that are well suited to them. The body, the skin, and the sense of touch are all arch conspirators in the formidable expression of the sexual human encounter. The significance of the noble body as a means of attraction to the opposite sex, and the exploratory powers of touch as the point of departure and prelude to an infinitely varied physical experience, has no counterpart in this world. It is an encounter that is dark and mysterious on the one hand, reaching down deep into the well of the human experience for the waters that reflect the sky far overhead, and most obvious and self-evident as a driving physical need on the other hand that no one needs further convincing about for we are all driven by its extravagant demands. In fact, who has the genuine insight, much less the right, to explore the dark intimacy that surrounds the physical sexual encounter between two people without shattering in some way the mythological and magisterial component of the experience? Does the interaction of the physical with our aesthetic and spiritual needs find its roots in the primitive and erotic subtext of our most primal instincts? Similarly, no one can pretend to escape from familiarity with the erotic and erogenous demands of sex upon the mind and the body, irrespective of the symbolic significance of the sex act in terms of the emotion of love that is the symbolic counterpart of the physical encounter. However, I will leave the opportunity to others who may be more inclined to explore the carnal and sensual side of the sexual encounter. Perhaps it is enough to know that the intimacy of love-making has a symbolic and ritualistic aspect whose depth and significance matches the intricate and incomparable intimacy that only two individuals left in privacy can explore and derive meaning from on their own.

❧

The human hand is a messenger of emotion that finds its expression in a variety of gestures and symbolic rituals. Even colloquial language uses the image of the hand to reach out with symbolic expressions that suggest a far deeper meaning. "I will give you a hand" actually means I will give you the best of myself, free willingly and without expectation of return. Hands are actually alive with meaning and emotion. They can be angry and accusatory as well as tender and expressive. Hands are perpetually in motion as expressions of inner moods, or they are silent and at rest, beautiful and elegant in repose. Hands can be the expression of abandonment as well as the reflection of awakening. There are criminal hands, artistic hands, tender hands, sick hands. In Islamic culture, the hand lying on the heart is the farewell expression of emotion and love at parting, while folded and cupped hands are the expression of supplication and repentance. Hands are like the source of some mighty river from which flows many expressions of life, pouring forth their abundance into the great stream of intention, desire, and action. Hands have beauty, history and art embodied with the five distinctive fingers, expressing their own feelings and moods and giving shape to a variety of artistic works that in being the expression of what is human are actually reflections of the Divine.

The holding of hands between two people can be the external expression of deeper reserves of friendship and love. I have three grandchildren who, when we set off together for a walk, fight for a place next to me to hold my hand and of course I have only two hands. When the baby Raouf takes my hand, it is with determination and love to hold on and never let go. His pudgy little paw grips several fingers as he holds on for dear life, and there is something sweet and incommunicable that passes between us by virtue of this physical connection, as though I was not holding his hand but the very essence of his soul in the form of a hand and thus had within my grasp a little piece of eternity. In many parts of the Islamic world, you can still find the close and bonding fraternal traditions that are usually associated with tribal life, where there are always very close connections between brothers, relatives and friends who constitute the greater familial network of the village. One of the first things that I noticed when I first came to the Middle East many years ago was the sight of two men walking along side by side holding hands. There was an attitude so frank and unassuming in the way they walked and talked that was incomprehensible to me at the time. Coming from the Western culture, the sight of two men holding hands came as a great surprise to me, leading me to wonder about the nature of the relationship. I soon learned how natural and spontaneous this hand-holding can be. In my experience, Arabs in general are much freer in their physical relationships, especially with other men since they essentially live in a social environment that encourages the separation of the sexes. They look you straight in the eye; they stand close to you; and they are not afraid to touch and be touched in return as the natural extension of gesture and communication. My good Pathan friend Farman sometimes takes my hand when we are walking down the street, and certainly if we are crossing a busy street, although the first time he took my hand like this, it felt like an electric current ran up my arm, so unaccustomed was I to this kind of casual and spontaneous expression of affection, if not protection. Eventually, I came to learn that in the touch of the extended hand there was a sort of clarity or purpose and a declaration of friendship and brotherhood that was physical as well as emotional and spiritual. There is nothing more spontaneous, fraternal and indeed sacred than in this physical connection of hands, arising as it does out of a natural feeling of affection and brotherhood. It reminds me of an interesting verse in the Quran: "The Hand of God is over your hands." (48:10) I have not know many men in the West who would dream of offering themselves so freely and openly through the symbolic gesture of holding someone's hand.

Just as we explore worlds within worlds through the sense faculties of sight and hearing, smell and taste; so also by touching others on some emotive or sympathetic plane, and being touched in return, we arrive at human experience that take us to another order of magnitude in terms of how we understand ourselves and our capacity to love humanity as a prelude to loving God. This is true of all touching between human beings, and it is significant that in the Islamic context Satan is said to lament whenever two Muslims shake hands. This simple physical contact between two human creatures is a token of the unity which Satan—the force of evil and disharmony—wishes to shatter. It is in accordance with the very nature of all symbolism that the most outward should reflect or express what is most profoundly inward and hidden. So, when I walk through wheat fields holding hands with my grandchild Raouf, or wander through the souk to do some shopping or make our way to the mosque for evening prayer and my friend Farman takes my hand, I know that I have arrived at an experience of touch that is a treasure beyond compare.

∽

The human hand and the subtle intricacies of the sense of touch also play a major role in the healing process. Their healing skill can be found in a variety of traditional massage techniques that go back thousands of years and find their roots in the sacred revelations of the various Far Eastern religions that still exist today in places like Thailand and Malaysia as a genuine form of alternative medicine. For example, there is an abundance of wisdom in the traditional knowledge contained within the sacred scriptures of the Vedanta. The medical science of Ayurveda that can be found faithfully practiced to this day in the South India state of Kerala has preserved a philosophy of medicine that focuses its applications on prevention and longevity in addition to the standard practices of healing and cure. It is in fact the oldest and most holistic medical system still available to modern humanity. What truly makes Ayurveda unique is its professed association with the spiritual tradition of a religion such as Hinduism. The knowledge itself has been transmitted to humanity through the divine revelation based on the four main books of the Vedas, including *Rik, Sama, Yajur* and *Atharva*. At later dates, the knowledge of Ayurveda was organized into its own compact system of health as an auxiliary branch of the Vedas called

Upaveda or "limb of the Veda", because it deals with the practical healing aspects within the realm of spirituality.

Using massage, internal herbal medicines, hot oils, cooling treatments, diet, life style, and a harmonious natural setting, Ayurveda leaves no stone unturned in coming to terms with the health and well being of a person. With its holistic philosophy of medicine based on traditional sources, Ayurveda uses everything within its means to affect a cure or better to achieve prevention of a disease affecting the body, mind, psyche, heart, or soul of the individual. All of these components interact in subtle ways of correspondence so that the disease or health of one aspect of the person necessarily affects some other aspect, and draws upon the principle of Supreme Unity that lies at the heart of the traditional doctrine of Hinduism as well as all of the other orthodox religions of the world. As such, Ayurveda draws upon everything that influences these various components that make up the human person, including massage, medicated oil, internal herbal medicines, heat treatments for certain diseases such as muscle and nerve problems, cooling treatments for arthritic problems and the like. As such, the importance of touch in the pursuit of these treatments plays a paramount role in affecting the cure.

Malaysia is another country that has faithfully preserved its tradition of massage as a legitimate means for affecting cure for many ailments such as muscle and nerve pain by addressing the medical problem at its source in order to bring about an effective cure. Anyone who has suffered the agonies of lower back pain will appreciate the unexpected encounter I had a number of years ago while I was working at a university in Kuala Lumpur. I had suffered for years from chronic lower back pain and it periodically came back to haunt me like an uninvited guest. It always arrived unannounced and stayed for months with an insistence that was hard to comprehend or ignore. The unbearable pain would be etched upon my face as stark evidence of my suffering. I would undergo every treatment under the sun from electric shock and heat treatments to ultrasound. After several months, the pain would eventually subside, but I was never truly convinced that it was the rarefied technological treatment, but rather sheer time that affected some kind relief and temporary cure until the pain would come back once again a year later.

One evening while drying my feet in the bathroom after a shower, I felt with impending dismay the old familiar stab of sciatica pain run down my body like a rip at the seam of my body. By the next morning, I could not turn around or lift myself from the bed. In desperation, I crawled to the telephone and called a Malay friend for help and advice. "Do you want to have a traditional massage," he asked me. "Why not," I replied, immediately receptive to such an intriguing offer? Of course, I had no real idea what he meant, but I was soon to find out.

As a group of villagers gathered to witness the unusual spectacle, my Malay friend Zainul-Din and several of his companions somberly carried me into the Malay kampong house, raised on stilts against invading insects, snakes and the inevitable tropical dampness. They wrapped me in a *batik* sarong and laid me on a floor mat on my back. The village elders sat down cross-legged around me and gazed meditatively and with concern at my supine body wracked in pain.

A traditional Malay masseur (called *dukun* in Malay) entered the room, and with quiet majesty knelt on his thighs by my side. He was a powerful-looking man for his modest size and advanced age, with clear skin and a round moon face that expressed the wisdom of his years. He put his thick, paw-like hands on my arm as if he were handling a dish rag. There was authority in his grip and a sense of presence to his touch that was distinctive and unmistakable. He solemnly asked my name in simple English, repeated it aloud, and made several invocations in Arabic which I later learned were epithets and verses from the Quran, used in order to actively invoke the presence of God into the proceedings. In truth, nothing happens in such traditional environments without first invoking the name of God in any event, a ritual that is still very prevalent within the Islamic community across the globe. Then he touched the palm of my hands with home-made herbal oil and proceeded to pressure point his way along my forearm from shoulder to wrist and back again.

There was no denying the pain generated by his powerful hands as he followed the line of muscle and nerve down my arm; it was excruciating, as if he were touching the raw nerve of my being. I cried out briefly while the group of villagers chatted and giggled nervously as they sat around and witnessed the proceedings. He worked on both arms and then moved down to the sides of the legs from hipbone to knee. The old Malay *dukun* radiated vitality and I could feel the power of his concentration and the force of his energy pass from his fingers into the tired and painful sinews of my body. He worked the muscles as though he were kneading dough and he could have been plucking the strings of a violin the way he pulled the meridians of muscles and nerve that run up and down the body back into their natural line of energy flow.

A vital aspect of the cure and one of its essential components is the encounter and relationship of the masseur affecting the cure and the person receiving the cure. It must be a relationship of complete acceptance and surrender, acceptance that the masseur has the ability and the power to bring about the cure through the power of the traditional laying on of hands as a medium of benediction and blessing, combined with the absolute surrender of the will of the person being treated with the body in a state of complete relaxation to the ministrations of the masseur. Without this interaction of complete connection and acceptance, no cure can be affected according to the traditional approach to healing.

Angin, the Malays call the problem, wind. On the physical plane, they believe that wind caused by many toxic elements including the icy cold drinks everyone loves accumulates in the body to ill effect. Indeed, as he proceeded with the massage, it did feel like wind as the pain shifted, diminished and ultimately disappeared under the pressure-pointing and stroking of his capable hands. Even the pain of the cure had a curative component that made the experience bearable to some degree. On another level, traditional Malays believe that devils—what are called *jinn* in the Islamic tradition— enter the body and set up residence to create havoc on physical, as well as psychic and spiritual levels. The notion is comparable to our beliefs concerning "possession" in which a person can be "possessed" by an evil spirit on mental or psychic levels.

Curiously, the masseur never actually touched my lower back; the pain was the final destination rather than the origin of the problem. Instead, he moved down and began to work his magic on the soles of my feet as if he were handling a rag doll. He began to knead and press against the muscles in the arch of one foot then the other with a focused stroke, causing an outrageous pain to run through me like a knife or some kind of electric shock to the system. He seemed to stop instinctively at some pain threshold of unbearability that held the promise of relief and healing. Still, I felt the need to give voice to my distress and I yelled like a banshee in fright and howled like a wolf in distress, much to the amusement of the villagers, curious about the identity of this *mate sale* (white devil in Malay). Throughout the ordeal, the *dukun* proceeded serenely with his work as if he were in some kind of otherworldly trance and periodically he would recite verses from the Quran or laughed to himself as I howled in outrage.

Malays are great talkers. My Malay friends and the other villagers carried on a running dialogue about the treatment, much of it in response to my questions. Such traditional masseurs believe in a holistic approach in which the interaction of both the physical and spiritual serve to affect the best possible cure. To that end, the masseur whispered a litany of Quranic incantations designed to raise the level of the experience and call upon the higher powers that be as protection against all evil. Finally, after an hour's worth of intense therapy, the old Malay sat back, indicating with a grunt that he was finished. A sublime feeling of relief surged through my body that was overwhelming and pure. I could hear in the distance the entreaties of the masseur to rest for a while before attempting to move. I lay quietly on my back seemingly in some kind of yoga trance and surrendered to a rare feeling of absolute peace that coursed through my body, as though a reservoir of well-being had been released in compensation for the outrage of the ordeal I had just endured.

Then, as suddenly and unexpectedly as a summer storm, from some deep well within me, there emerged the inexplicable urge to cry. The source of this impulse was completely unknown to me although its impending presence was real enough. To my shock and amazement, I then began to weep aloud, first quietly, then in great choking sobs that shook my whole body in embarrassing spasms, although the origin of this emotion remained a mystery to me, leading me to wonder who within me was crying in this way and why, as though some other voice had taken possession of me and wanted to give expression of some sort. I had the feeling not I, but something inside me was giving voice to a terrible sadness. Perplexed, I let myself go and surrendered to the experience with curiosity and detachment, as I watched myself cry my heart out, with real tears.

The great heartbreaking sobs eventually subsided as I shook myself free from the grip of some uncontrollable experience and I was once again calm enough to inquire what had happened, for I could not understand or explain the reason for my outburst. 'It was the *jinn*,' my friend Zainul-din told me. 'Whatever do you mean?' I asked incredulous. 'The bad *jinn* are reluctant to leave the body and cry out loud when forced to do so,' he replied casually. Improbable as it sounded, I was not in a position to counter his theory with an explanation of my own. In any event, I was suddenly summoned by the old *dukun* to rise from the bamboo mat. He indicated with gestures to bend forward and backward, then to stand up altogether and walk around the room. I looked at him in surprise as he smiled knowingly. The outrageous pain that I had suffered for weeks, indeed for years, had completely disappeared.

Was it the rare communion of body, mind, and spirit culminating in an experience of healing that seems alien to the realities of the modern world? Was it a foreign presence as suggested, not of alien beings from outer space but rather evil spirits from an inner space with the capacity to transform well-being into chronic and debilitating pain? Malays, indeed many Muslims, are fond of saying when they are confronted with some inexplicable mystery: 'Only God knows!' As for myself, while I had been carried into the village house like a sick lamb, there was no denying the special light of this unexpected encounter and miraculous cure that shone down upon me that day. I expressed profound gratitude and with feelings of humility took my leave of the old Malay masseur, walking out of the house and into the wilds of the jungle village on the strength of my own two feet, feeling that I had been touch by more than two aged hands; indeed I was touched by a benediction and a mercy that was invisible to behold.

We referred earlier to infant children as poets and visionaries because their sense of wonder, joy and imagination is as raw, pure, primitive and uncorrupted as the spiritual intuitions that are their natural inheritance of the timelessness they come from. Poets, on the other hand, find magical and visionary meaning in outward forms. They reach out and touch as it were the artifacts of nature as living, breathing entities that are symbolic and full with meaning, archetypal symbols whose energy and rhythms echo higher realities, and like the natural beauties of nature, the spiritual poems they create breathe in the life they represent, glow in the dark, and speak directly to the heart. This is what the poet gives voice to, and in doing so reaches out and touches the mind and hearts of those who partake of their verses. In their exploration of the meaning of the natural order, they continually roam across the frontier of the great open spaces where the Divinity can be found. A dew drop falling from a blade of grass may create an exquisite sense of rapture; the rustle of the wind through the trees a momentary cataclysm of insight. In reaching out with the fingers of the mind to touch some forgotten reality and to be touched in return, they discover frontiers that reaffirm the pristine, if evanescent, nature of the world.

Think of the romantic poets and Robert Burns comes to mind, whose love is "like a red, red rose that's newly sprung in June". Born of a flight of imaginative fancy, these dreamy images find their basis in sensuous facts, at a safe distance from the deep well of a latent and far more profound human experience. Sacred poetry, on the other hand, draws upon a super-sensual wealth of symbolic images that abound in nature, allowing the sun, moon and stars and the world of nature they drench their light upon to send messages of extraordinary beauty and depth to the sensibility of the poet who stands and waits to become the transmitter of their rich, subtle mystery. As a medium of a deeper and more revelatory communication from the human to the Divine, the verses of spiritual poetry give expression to the eternity out of which they are born. In this sense, the poets themselves become a part of the eternity they drew upon; they cannot die.

Indeed poets still exercise their imagination and intuitive powers to touch and inspire people with a spiritual message that transcends time and the generations. People who pick up an anthology of spiritual poetry and peruse its contents will be opening the door of their heart to an unexpected awakening. There is a poet in every one of us by virtue of the human capacity not only to respond to the symbolic language that poetry draws upon, but to feel the sudden inrush and be touched by some experience vaster than ourselves coming as though from another world and another self. As the compendium and conduit of a hidden message cast within beautiful linguistic forms and echoing the natural cadences of rhythm and rhyme whose harmonies trace their origin back to God, the music of poetry lends wings to the reader and transports them higher and farther than they could ever imagine on their own. "Ah, no wings of the body could compare to wings of the spirit! It is in each of us inborn.[2]

Spiritual poetry are soul songs, giving birth to a fearless, soaring progeny that reflects the beauty of the poet's soul across a broad spectrum of spiritual traditions. The mysterious tone of the koto[3] echoes an unearthly sound "from within my own breast"; our earthly fears are "among the lilies fading"; my heart, taking any and every form, becomes "a pasture of gazelles" and a "pilgrim's Kaaba"; we have within us the "singing flute that came from the sea"; we learn to die "in time", while Time will die "in eternity".[4] Only in the ethereal realms of such mystical poetry can we become as Bedouin tent-makers in some desert clime where the body is called "a tent" and the soul "a sultan from the eternal world". The poet sings intuitively and wildly, turning the evanescence of misty clouds into flowers of the mind and heart. Why shouldn't thoughts and impressions that are strange and beautiful and true to the poet resonate their harmonies within the soul of the reader so they too can participate in the sublime messages of nature? In compensation, perhaps

---

2. Goethe, as quoted in Theodore Roszak's *Where the Wasteland Ends*, p. 346.

3. A kind of zither that has been used as one of the main chamber instruments of Japanese traditional music style.

4. Poetry quotations cited here are taken from the book *Music of the Sky*, ed. Barry MacDonald (Bloomington, IN: World Wisdom Books, 2005).

nature's peace will shine its mercy down upon all earthlings and flow into their aspiring soul as sunshine flows into trees.

Spiritual and mystic poems reflect the outpourings of an open soul, poems for the ages that transcend their own boundaries with their unique spiritual messages and seem to the reader like drinking cool water from a hand-carved wooden bowl. The poems appear out of nowhere like a field of wild lilies, unruly and joyous, shouting insights into our sullen modern minds like magical incantations from another age for anyone and everyone to listen to and behold. Their music seems to fall from the sky, and is evocative of a higher order of consciousness and experience, linking the implicit music of verse with the harmonies and rhythms evidenced through the universe, while the image of the sky recalls the broad sweep of the Infinite contained within that plate of empyrean blue. The externalization of such sublime thought through sound and word images becomes internalized as an inner harmony within the firmament of the human soul and spirit.

Poetry has something to say that cannot strictly be put into words, similar to the verses of revelation which contain levels of knowledge that cannot be contained by the form of the words alone; there is always hidden meaning belonging to some higher plane that will actually reveal itself to the receptive soul. As such, it is less subjective and more objective in the sense that the words and images of the poem convey a meaning that finds its root in the Divine Reality. In this sense, poetic recitation produces an uncanny emotion within the individual that could be called "an objective emotion"; an emotion insofar as a spiritual sentiment moves the heart and 'objective' insofar as the emotion is grounded in a divine archetype amounting to the "true nature" of a given phenomenon.

Succinct and summative are the traditional symbols that shake the cords of the heart and shatter the foundation of the soul, especially modernite souls of today made complacent and dull by the false promises that underpin the modern world. When a poet such as Rumi cries "We are the flute, our music is all thine; We are the mountains echoing only Thee", we come to understand that we are not ourselves, that there are elements in nature such as the wind whispering through the pines or the echo of a distant flute that have qualities that remind us of the best of ourselves and have the power to transport us to other worlds by the very suggestion of their sounds. When we learn that "poor Yunus fills the earth and sky, and under every stone hides a Moses," it reminds the unwary reader that we may be more than we make ourselves out to be, that there is a living presence within us that makes us what we are, that there is greatness awaiting discovery. The images abound, unrelenting and incisive, that for sheer splendor create a diversity of forms that unite under no true difference. What is the world but "moonlight reflected in dewdrops"; who is standing there "divinely dignified" but the solitary pine tree; the desires of a human life is reflected in the sockets of "his earthly lanthorn" and that all life's glory "unto ashes must". Rain "whispers of reality" to an obliging ear; fog arrives "like a spring dream" and departs "like the morning clouds" and there is no way to own these things. Nature calls us to remembrance, sweetly and insistently, and then leaves us on our own as it passes us by.

As a purely human phenomenon, spiritual poetry are songs of the heart because they attempt to express the ineffable sentiments that emerge from some secret niche or cave within the human being where the kingdom of God resides "within you". As the individual expression of the poet's most heart-felt yearning, it becomes the human kingdom with the power not only to imagine, but also to feel the knowledge of God as a living presence. A poet lies secreted within every one of us by virtue of the human capacity not only to see the inner reality, but to internalize the true meaning of that reality through symbolic language. It is as if a piece of the heavens has come down to us in the form of heart songs of the poets and spiritual masters of a former time, revisited during these post-modern times as votive candles in the deepening dusk of the present era. In a sense, spiritual poems open the heart to a rude awakening of what we have become, conveying a sense of nostalgia for the higher consciousness and loss of the sense of the Presence that we have lost during these times.

The mystic poet is a person with the power to quicken the heart because his own heart has awakened to the realm of pure feeling. He traverses whole realms of experience of which other people only dream. Many spiritual poems are extraordinarily short, concise, and sharp as a knife-blade. Indeed who can say that a poem need be long when in fact there was once a time when every word was itself a kind of poem. The writers of spiritual poetry are sacred image makers one and all. They give a thing a name because they come one step nearer to perceiving something more than any other person who passes the same way. They look out into the world of nature and see that between human nature and earthly nature there is one interlocking thread binding them as a single unity. In highlighting the archetypal meaning of the symbol, the poet doesn't give entrance into a land of hidden meaning; instead the sacred symbols of nature and the meaning they contain enter us, lending of their mystery and grace to become the persons we once were in principle and are still meant to be in fact. They are poems written one from heart to another heart with no boundaries or intermediaries, creating a place where people can roam freely by virtue of the participation in the land of the poem itself.

On our own, we do not sufficiently address ourselves to the clues and signals that life has to offer in terms not only of life's implicit mystery, but also its hidden disclosure. Our work and efforts, our politics and prejudices, our false morality and pseudo truths, our shallow imaginations and empty satisfactions, our hollow words and feeble aspirations will all go unsung across the generations because they are unworthy of our true attentions and unfit as the stuff of our heart's desire. Images of the old master sitting, "a rock, in Zen" and the desire to live to see "in huts and on journeys the great day that dawns" are specters of the eternal because they contain an eternal ethos that lives forever as truth and comes down into the realm of the earthly as a sweet remembrance of a higher order. We are the "lattices" in the niche of time "through which the One Light shines." Few men and women ever perceive these things on their own; they rely on the largeness of mind and wisdom of the poet who sees the archetypes of the grand order fall down into the symbolic images of nature and humankind filling forms with other-worldly meaning. We cannot escape the world; not many people want to these days. But we can take leave of the world for a few moments through the rarefied perceptions and noble dignity conveyed through these seed-words of the soul, representing an outpouring from the sacred ground of the heart, and an inpouring into the sacred ground of the soul.

The magnificent beauty of the creation is matched by the sublime miracle of consciousness. Within Nature, the voice of thunder peels across the firmament, the sound of the wind whispers through the pine trees, the dawn mist creeps silently through the valley, night and day chronicle the procession of time. These features of the Divinity outlined within the phenomenal world and etched upon the mind of the true poet as mental icons that convey a meaning that can never be fully expressed in words. Wherever snow falls or birds fly, whenever the river flows into the sea, whenever the seasons change or twilight descends into darkness, the poet captures these images in seed words of beauty and light as a remembrance of an omnipresent order of Reality that lifts us up and takes us away, out into the open sky, where the vision of the one Reality has freedom to roam and the sound of the eternal music sends forth its celestial harmonies until their richness comes down to earth and touches human ears.

～

We have explored the role and significance of the sense of touch as a talisman between the human body and the world and between two individuals. We have seen the world as a bridge between the physical and the metaphysical, between the visible and invisible, and between the audible and inaudible, while the five senses, for all of their functionality and subtlety, are but instruments, water-carriers, donkeys to bear the burden of the world beyond its logical conse-quence into the realm of sheer mystery. We have reflected upon the curative powers of touch through the energy and life force of the hands and we have ventured forth into the visionary world of spiri-tual poetry that transcends the sensory delights of nature found in bird song, flower smell, sky color and herb taste for the beatitudes of the paradise through the language of men posing as angels, reaching out and bringing forth symbols and mysteries and inspira-tions that pass from the inspired poet to the poetic and intuitive mind of the reader.

However, the sense of touch reaches out and experiences its most tender and heart-felt moment, not between humanity and the world, not from one person to another, and not from the artist and visionary to a receptive audience in search of enlightenment, but between human yearning and the Divine promise, between surrender and unity. The Prophet used to say: "O God, let there be in my heart light, and in my hearing light, and in my seeing light, in my hands light, to my right light, to my left light, and let me be light." According to a famous verse of the Quran: "Allah is the Light of the Heavens and the Earth."

We wear ourselves like a suit of clothes, punishing our physical bodies with an excess of sensations; we make our way through the world like blind men feeling for signposts along the way; we reach out in love and affection to substantiate our desires and to express our heart-felt yearnings for our loved ones. But what of the Beloved, the universal object of all true desire, the One who sees (*al-Basir*) and the One who listens (*al-Samir*)? What about the supreme Friend upon which the entire narrative of humanity is based? Is there an inner meaning to the sense of touch that transcends the mundane world of physical objects and even the emotive world of human hearts reaching out to touch one another? Is there a final emotion that sweeps away all desire and lays us bare, a *tabula rasa*, naked and virgin, to the primitive and universal instincts that have us reach beyond ourselves, beyond our own ragged edges, and beyond the event horizon of the universe, to write upon the surface of our being through a calligraphy of worship and love the knowledge of the universal truth of one Reality.

All of the spiritual modes of worship, including prayer and Quranic recitation, can create a focused frame of mind and a conducive atmosphere of spirituality that fully supports the proposed encounter and communication with God, the mantra through the sheer effect of primordial sound, the sacred formula of the *shahadah* (testament of faith in Islam) through its quintessential and revealed knowledge, prayer through its personal and heart-felt aspiration as a channel of spiritual communication and human sentiment, and scriptural recitation as a sacred science and sonoral art whose intimate and transcending function relates directly to the form and content of the revelation itself, making available to the faithful its inner reality and its sacramental presence.

There remains yet another aspect of worship in the form of deep prayer that devotees within the Islamic perspective have perpetuated as a meditative invocation of the Name that begins in quietude and darkness and comes to fruition as an experience of sonorous harmony and spiritual enlightenment. According to Ali, the fourth Caliph of Islam, "Silence is the garden of meditation." Traditional meditation and the invocation of the holy Name represent intense forms of worship that create a heightened focus and powerful ambiance that raises the level of spiritual consciousness to another order of spirituality once it is truly felt. Individual prayer operates on the transpersonal level with its subjective and votive aspects emerging out of the individual's need to express a personalized spiritual emotion. Canonical prayer operates on the more formal level of ritual with its impersonal and universal aspect that draws directly on the cosmic sources of knowledge and grace. Meditation operates on the purely interior level with an objective and absolute aspect that rests in full contemplation of Knowledge as Truth and Divinity as Presence. Invocation operates on the repetitive level of remembrance with its sole emphasis on the revealed Name of God as the passageway leading toward unity with the Divine Being.

Both meditation and invocation awaken an experience of profound introspection that neutralizes the human ego through a forgetting of the self in order to discover and experience a level of consciousness that has the potential to reach a higher level of spirituality for the soul. Both of these modes of spiritual discipline can produce a great levelling of the personal ego, together with the exclusion of all the images of the self and the world, in order to create a "mindlessness" that is characterized by such a supra-consciousness and a clarity that is paradoxically characteristic of a certain kind of wakefulness that quiets the mind and softens the heart for contemplation on the "one things essential", and ultimately soothes the entire being into a trance of serenity and peace, recalling the saying: "I sleep, but my heart awakens."

All the major, orthodox religious traditions, including Taoism, Hinduism, Buddhism, Christianity and Islam, encourage modes of meditation and invocation as the most profound avenue available to humanity of spiritual expression into the deeper spiritual realities as a means of drawing near to God in this world as a prelude and foretaste of the paradisal plenitude. Because they are formless and universal in their approach, there is a commonality of purpose behind these spiritual disciplines that includes a levelling of the ego, a fundamental forgetting of the self, a systematic pursuit of interiorization, an attempt to pierce through the illusions of the mind and heart, a focusing of consciousness through centering postures and breathing techniques that enable the practitioner to see and understand everything in a wider framework and context by focusing on the natural rhythms of breathing and on the human heart through the pulse. The repetition of one of the sacred names, or the Name of names for that matter, stimulates the spiritual imagination which in turn predisposes the heart and prepares the ground of the soul to become receptive to the divine Light. The ambience of silence created, which Ali, the companion of the Prophet and fourth caliph, has called "the garden of meditation", is characterized by a focused silence complemented by an inner stillness, characteristics that are manifested in every religious tradition, silence because it shuts out the cacophony of "this world" including the external world of dispersion and heaviness and the inner world of thoughts, desires, anxieties, and illusions, and stillness because it represents the inner calm and absolute serenity that must characterized the perfection of the Paradise and the harmony that can result from an honest attempt to communicate with the Divine Reality. "Call Me and I will answer you," the Quran reassures the faithful.

The practice of *dhikr* or holy invocation of the Name of Allah in perpetual remembrance is not for everyone; just as it is not for everyone to go jungle-trekking through the tropical forests of the Far East. There is a wild and uncompromising spirit, unburdened by thought and book learning, waiting across some vast chasm between the visible and the invisible, an ancient presence waiting to be approached that contains all the pasts and futures that anyone could ever want, a presence that only needs to be acknowledged and thus to be touched in order to reveal the eternal moment within the present tense of our lives. Just as one experiences something strange and unique upon entering a primitive tropical forest, there is an overwhelming sense of wild and primitive nature within the human mind to the extent that one must become wild and unfettered and free of the fear that might otherwise overtake the mind in such an alien and powerful setting that lies within us like a jungle. In return there is the promise of a wild joy awaiting those who bridge the gap between the known and the unknown.

I worked for a number of years in Alexandria, Egypt as a teacher at a local university. The most notable thing that I remember from that experience, and will always remember, is the extent of the devotion and love that my Egyptian students showered upon me without asking anything in return. They would surround me after class with comments and questions to the point of exasperation. When I left the classroom and made my way out into the warm Egyptian night, they followed me with their animated chatter, follow me all the way to the tram stop and entertain me while I was waiting for the tram with their incessant joking and their infectious laughter. When the tram eventually rumbled by, I attempt to take my leave with muted *salaams*; but they would have nothing of it and would climb aboard the tram with me until the time came when I would have to "descend" as they say in Arabic and get off at my stop. Sure enough, they followed me with their questions and laughter and led me all the way to my door, at which point, I shook their hands and disappeared into the inner sanctum of my apartment, leaving in my wake the happy chatter of my students as they made their way home to their crowded, dingy flats.

After the sunset prayer one evening at a local mosque, I was approached by a small gathering of young Egyptians who were curious and interested to learn my "story", how did it come about that they found me in the mosque, as if I were one of them. They soon learned that I was Muslim and had been Muslim for many years, having converted to Islam probably before many of them were even born. I was introduced to one of the Sufi Sheikhs of the area and was made to feel welcome at his Thursday night gatherings.[5] The sheikh himself was well educated and had a magnetic personality

5. The Islamic day begins at sunset, so technically speaking the gathering on Thursday evening had significance in that it was already Friday, the day of congregation when the Muslims gather *en masse* for the Friday noon prayer.

that drew a person into the glow of his sanctified aura. It wasn't sur-prising to learn that he had a huge following, many of whom would gather together with the sheikh for the Thursday night *dhikr* session that was the hallmark of the evening. There was never any plan or program, no announcements and no encouragement to attend these gatherings. Given my Western upbringing, the sheikh made it clear that he wanted me to attend, if for no other reason than to make me feel welcome. In fact, between the sheikh and his beloved followers, they all made it clear that they extended every love and consideration to me while I was there in attendance. Their love for me was spontaneous and freely given; my love for them was initially responsive and in reflection of their own heart-felt sentiments. Egyptians are very social people and they have great respect for for-eigners. This was during the time of Sadat when there was great rapprochement between Egypt and the US in the wake of the Camp David agreement. Needless to say, every Egyptian's dream was to find himself in America to take part in what they considered the great American dream. Of course to them, I was a Muslim first and then an American as an added advantage, guaranteed to enter Para-dise, they loved to tell me, by virtue of having converted to Islam of my own free will. "You are better than us," they loved to say.

The sheikh had a large apartment and it is part of the domestic Islamic culture not to clutter rooms with excessive furniture and not to hang things such as pictures or artwork on the walls as deco-ration, the one exception being the occasional hanging of Quranic verses on the walls of a room or sacred Islamic art such as Quranic calligraphy. At a signal from the sheikh, the large gathering of young, middle aged, and elderly people dressed in Egyptian jall-abiyahs[6] moved into a second, larger room and formed a grand cir-cle standing with everyone holding hands, the sheikh taking up his central position within the group. For a few moments, there was a hushed silence, a kind of sacred anticipation if you will, in which all the negative energy of life seemed to drain away from the group

---

6. The Egyptian full length and flowing jallabiyah being a dead give-away that a person was from the nearby villages and were peasants or farmers, called *fallaheen* in Arabic.

together with a letting go or surrender if you will, the noise and distraction of the world falling by the wayside. It felt like a collective pause, as if the group had taken a deep breath and had neglected to exhale, or perhaps purposefully held the spirit of the breath within themselves in anticipation of the sacred ritual that was about to begin. The sheikh commenced the session by intoning certain sacred epithets from the Quran and these phrases were quickly taken up with rhythmic resonance by the large circle of initiates.

Immediately, the room became transformed into sacred space echoing in abundance the waves of sacred sound. The circle of devotees held each other's hands and rhythmically began chanting the supreme Name of Allah while bending their knees and rocking their bodies back and forth. I could see the white skull caps of the faithful as they bent their heads, and the flowing multi-colored kaftans of the older sheikhs fluttered like banners in the turmoil of the wind, created by the collective movement of the group. I felt at one with the multitude as we intoned the Name Allah in repeated inflections in a rising crescendo of sacred psalmody, my own body and mind at one with the bodies rocking back and forth in the darkness of the night. There was a rising tide of sound in the room that was impossible to countermand as the voices of what seemed like a thousand men uttered the name of God again and again in ritual repetition, forming a solemn intonement that was hypnotizing. We in the West have completely forgotten that repeating a divine name over and over is tantamount to identifying oneself with this name and consequently with God Himself.[7] It was as if the floor shook under our feet and my legs felt as weak as rubber. The sheikh himself worked the circle as though not wishing to neglect anyone and leaving no one alone, passing in front of each one of the devotees with his right hand raised in the air, pointing with his index finger in tribute to the great witnessing of the *shahadah* or sacred formula in Islam.[8] As

7. Ramahrishna has said: "God and His name are identical." The Sufis have said: "God is present in His Name."

8. After the bowing and prostrations of the prayer ritual, the Muslims silently intone the *shahadah* and at the same moment raise the index finger of the right hand as a symbolic gesture affirming faith in God.

he stood in front of me, I could feel his presence even though I had my eyes closed. The sheikh radiated a holy presence that seemed to sparkle and I could feel the power of his love enter my soul, mingling with my own heightened emotions as they rose back up to God, who was in truth the object of true desire for the multitude of worshippers in the room.

One hour, two hours, time went by as though in an instant, for the continuum of time has no true framework to capture this kind of experience within its mundane embrace. At times, I felt as though I was being lifted on high off the ground, the rhythm and resonance of the sacred name was so resounding and so powerful. It seemed as though a thousand echoes were making their way to some invisible shore on a tide of sound, at other times it sounded like muted cloth that unfurled like banners in the wind blowing in the direction of some distant horizon in search of fulfilment in the mythical realm of "beyond".

There were those who faltered and lost their breath; one person fainted; several others fell to the floor only to be helped back up by the ever vigilant sheikh who scrupulously watched over his flock and would let no one wander away either physically or mentally. The rhythm became breathless and the clarity of the sound united into some primitive, primal force that was indistinguishable from the proto-language (*Ursprache*) of the Divinity. Eyes were shut and voices became hoarse; there were tears in the night. I do not know whether it was the collective emotion of the horde or some secret door from within that had finally opened, but I felt a sudden rush of emotion and tears floods my eyes and fell down my checks as I sank into a deep emotive well of abandonment and lack of caring of all that I thought I loved, my friends, my job, my money, my books, my writing, my successes in life such as they were. It seemed like some great sense of love was being born out of the chrysalis of my former self as an exquisite butterfly, or as though a diamond-shaped crystal was beginning to emerge out of the lodestone of the heart. Something indefinable was being created approximating the feeling of limitless love that seemed to ride on the intonation of the sacred name as the name of the Beloved. There was a feeling of intoxication to the experience that was undeniable, fused by the true spirit of the moment that brought the Infinite and the Eternal down into temporal time for one brief spellbound encounter with the holy Presence that was unmistakable because it was truly experienced.

Whether I had stepped across an invisible threshold or fallen off the edge of some symbolic horizon denoting the limits of "this world", there was an overwhelming sensation of having arrived at the open spaces of a boundless frontier whose horizon blended into the heavens in a seamless unity. A boundless spiritual freedom filled the room that was there for the taking and perpetuated by the swirling vortex of the sheikh driving us forward with his compelling spiritual force—a vibrant, joyous freedom that rose up into the mind like the vaulted dome of a grand mosque, vaulted to the skies and reaching heavenward with its enveloping bliss. It was as though we were caught to a man in a powerful embrace and were drowning in the wavelets of a universal sound that embodied the name of God and that cleared the way to His Presence.

I remember thinking at some point: I am a ball of yarn unraveling, wondering what lie within the center of this disappearing universe, unraveling slowly but surely with every resonant sound. There was a distinct feeling of letting go and giving something up, something that once given up would set you free. We sometimes have a similar sensation when we dream during the slumber of the night. Falling asleep is a letting go of sorts and a giving up of the active consciousness. There is the presumption of trust that in falling asleep, we will once again awaken. If we dream, there is the sense of a temporary freedom in the timelessness of the dream and provided it isn't a nightmare, the dream state can be extremely liberating. The *dhikr* or oral remembrance of God is a letting go of the self in search of union with the Supreme Self. In roaming through the inner world of darkness behind closed eyes, I began to see some inner world of light. A small point of illumination made its way through the darkness of my mind to become a swirling and multicolored spiral of iridescence, like a spinning sun with phosphorescent trails of light, undulating in the darkness like a living animal. I opened my eyes at one point, to replace the darkness behind my eyelids with the darkness of the room, but that spinning spiral of light continue to pulsate in the darkness, turning into the vision of a million fire flies that was alarming to behold, a light that one could loose oneself seemingly, forever.

The profundity of the moment was so simple really; no one could deny the truth of the experience. You reach out through revelation and spiritual discipline; you engage the entire body in ritual movements that heighten the experience of the moment; you use the sound of your voice to call down through invocation and remembrance the sacred sound of revelation that is witnessed by the angels, when behold, the very *sakinah* or supreme peace descends into the souls of the devotees. And nothing and no one could stand in its way, not even ourselves.

Some time later, the sheikh slowed down the rhythm of the multitude, brought the shouts and exclamations of the worshippers down to a whisper that soon drifted off into the night as the lights came back on in the empty darkened room. How long had we been entranced with the remembrance of the Name no one could tell you or even cared to wonder. The sheikh's followers embraced and kiss one another with bright light on their faces and with gestures of deep fraternity that they felt for one another. I was of course included in the embrace of these great bear hugs and felt at one with this rarefied community of friends. We sat down on the carpet and tea was served in miniature cups, clear golden tea that tasted like the nectar of the paradise.

⌒

The Quran and *hadith* abound with references to the *dhikr* or remembrance of God. There are verses and sayings of the Prophet that attest to its vital importance to the believer in his pursuit of spirituality. We have already mentioned the well-known Quranic verse (29:45) "Establish prayer, but remembrance is the greatest thing." Also the definitive statement on remembrance: "Remember Me, and I will remember you" (or "Mention Me and I will mention you" [2:152]). In fact, remembrance plays such a major role in the return to God that the Prophet of Islam is also recorded as saying: "All in the world is accursed except the remembrance of God." The hyperbole may seem a little strong, but so also is the importance of the remembrance of God in the life of man, important enough that in truth, nothing else matters or would matter if a person truly had the God-consciousness that is the direct consequence of the remembrance (*dhikr*). "God guides to Him ... those who believe and whose hearts are at rest in God's remembrance because surely, in God's remembrance are hearts at rest" (13:27–28).

Invocation of the Holy Name offers the believer three distinct blessings. It is a form of divine remembrance that actually raises the level of human consciousness to the threshold of the heavenly spheres and ultimately the very presence of God. After a brief session involving the invocation of the sacred Name, the invoker quite literally takes the effects of this heightened consciousness back out into the world with him, altering in shades of light and degrees of perception his very understanding of the world with this overlay of divine remembrance. Secondly, invocation of the Name provides the ultimate means of opening the door of the human mind with the vertical perception which is none other than a means of discrimination that permits the person who is meditating to experience the spiritual realities as a human reality. Thirdly, invocation of the sacred Name contains spiritual energy within its very sonoral and auditory form that strikes the human entity with a shower of blessing and grace like stardust from a celestial wand. These blessings are a holy by-product of the efforts implicit in this form of supererogatory worship. They infiltrate the mind and heart of the believer with feelings of confidence, inner contentment, tranquillity, happiness and peace, in short with those very gifts that man innerly yearns for at the root of his being. Needless to say, the ultimate gift of Heaven is the truth of certainty (*al-haqq al-yaqin*) which negates all doubt within the heart and places man at the disposition of his own sacred center with all the force of his free will.

The Prophet himself stressed the importance of the invocation as the remembrance *par excellence* for the faithful. "Shall I tell you the best of your deeds? The purest in the eyes of your King, He whom you hold to be at the highest level, Whose proximity is more beneficial than the act of giving gold and silver or of meeting your enemy and striking him down or being struck?" The companions of the Prophet said, "Tell us." The Prophet answered, "It is the invocation of God the Most High." Another well known tradition reports the Prophet as saying: "There is a way of polishing everything and removing rust and that which polishes the heart is the invocation of God." Another saying states through hyperbole[9] the fundamental importance of this spiritual practice: "An hour of meditation is better than sixty years of acts of worship." And finally: "Men never assemble to invoke Allah without being surrounded by angels and covered by Divine Blessings, and without peace (*sakinah*) descending on them and Allah remembering them."

The holy invocation of the Name *Allah* can be seen as operative on three different levels, levels that correspond with the three levels of the religion, namely that of the law (*shari'ah*), which establishes the doctrinal infrastructure of the religion, the way (*tariqah*) which provides an inner focus and a clear direction, and the truth (*haqiqah*) which represents the absolute authority and final word in the human narrative. Firstly, there is the invocation of the tongue (*dhikr al-lisan*) which is the very gift of speech that distinguishes man from the animals and that is the outward form of sound that verbalizes the substance of the inner consciousness. Invocation through auditory sound with its hypnotic inner focus unites all aspects of man into a single totality focused on none other than the Divinity through the Name. Secondly, there is the invocation of the heart (*dhikr al-qalb*) that focuses the mind and the consciousness on the human center of the heart, out of which flows the knowledge and love of God, the heart being the seat of the intelligence as well as the fountain of all humanly spiritual sentiment. Finally, the invocation emerges from the very core of the heart, the heart of hearts and blessed center (*dhikr al-sirr*) as it were and the place where tears are

---

9. It should be pointed out especially to a Western readership that Arab style prefers, and the Arab mentality appreciates, the use of hyperbole among other figures of speech. Hyperbole works for the Arab mind because it appreciates the essence first and foremost, even at the expense of the form of a thing. In an expression such as this one, in which the value of meditation is equated to sixty years of worship, it is the intention and meaning behind the words that count and not the literal estimation of a sixty year time period. The hyperbole is used to convey a basic truth in a spiritually emotive manner and not to convey a literal truth in a cold, matter of fact manner.

stored, that contains the human secret as a reflection of the Divine Mystery. Through repetition and invocation of the sacred Name, the invoker denies everything and affirms nothing, except the One God who through the efficacy of the sacred Name is the One called upon and the One invoked.

The final emotion that we all instinctive seek by virtue of the inner sense of touch, so beautifully symbolized in Michelangelo's painting on the ceiling of the Sistine Chapel in which the great artist depicts the fingertips of the human and the Divine reaching out toward each other in profound yearning on the eternal Day, is not easily achieved. The answer lies in the preservation of spiritual disciplines and practices within the routine of our lives. Spiritual practices assume many forms of human expression, but all aspire to one single end: To cross through modes of worship and praise the unbreachable isthmus that exists between human and divine worlds in order to establish a communication with the Divinity, an earthly encounter that anticipates the union of the human soul with the Spirit of God in Paradise.

Behind the sense of touch lies a spirit waiting to unfold, just as beneath the placid surface of life flows a revolutionary current coursing through our bodies, through the world, through the universe. In reaching out to touch the pulse of life, whether it be in the form of a child's penetrating gaze, a healing hand, a poet's fabled imagery, or the heart-felt yearning and love of the aspiring soul through spiritual practices, we are reaching for that invisible and non-tangible reality that escapes the scrutiny of the outer senses, but that manifests itself through their implicit wisdom, revealing knowledge and light that is dazzling to behold, "gleaming", in the words of the romantic poet Blake, "like the flashing of a shield."[10]

Do we turn to the God who created us, much less invoke His name and take part in His sweet remembrance? Is the active consciousness of the Reality but a distant memory of earlier peoples, preserved like a dried flower in a book and hidden away in a drawer under freshly ironed handkerchiefs as a hidden treasure awaiting some providential discovery. On the Day of Judgment, every resur-

10. Theodore, Roszak, *Where the Wasteland Ends.*

rected soul will be asked to give an accounting of their thoughts and actions during their lifetime. Who will be prepared on that momentous occasion to confess to the gathered multitude that they had neglected "the one thing needful" and forgotten the truths that could be found under every rock and blade of grass? Happy indeed will be those who took the time to remember the Divinity by reaching out with their mind and heart toward the Spirit of God. In compensation for their efforts, they will be remembered in return.

Call upon Me and I will remember you. (Quran)

7

THE INTUITIVE POWER
OF THE SIXTH SENSE

One searched in vain beyond phenomenon;
it in itself is revelation.'
(Goethe)

In addition to the blessings of the five senses, with their exotic sights
and sounds, and their aromatic smells and tastes, not to mention
the sublime sensation of touch that sears the flesh and lifts the heart
out of its cage, there lies in waiting another, unidentified sense that
garners information without the use of reason and gathers knowledge without using the formal instruments of perception at the disposal of human ingenuity. We are in principle sentient creatures[1]
that, because of our status as conscious beings, have the capacity to
know without seeing, to perceive without hearing, to understand
without smelling or tasting, and to feel without actually touching a
thing. The question remains: how is this accomplished and what is
the agency through which the miraculous becomes manifest to the
human mentality? What has the capacity to open our minds and
hearts to the "other side" of reality?

There is a point beyond which the five senses cannot lead us,
but having arrived at this outer edge of experience and point of no
return, we have only to take one further step in order to cross the
threshold from outer perception to inner experience. We have
suggested in earlier chapters that there is an inner realm that is

---

1. From the Latin *sentire*, 'to feel'.

enclosed within the outer world that complements its experience, so that in smelling perfume and incense we are lifted beyond the limits of the experience to a higher place of consciousness. We need to complete the narrative of this untold story by suggesting that there is a faculty of knowledge and perception, a sixth sense in common parlance, that is an operative faculty in the same way that the five senses are operative instruments of perception, with the power to open doors and raise spirits to a level of experience that would be unimaginable to the human mentality on its own.

We say that there are five senses for the sake of convenience; yet we know that there is more to these tools than meets the eye that aid both animals and humans in negotiating their way through the intricacies of the world. Bats see in the night through sophisticated echo sounds and birds migrate across great distances through memory and instinct. Butterflies and whales navigate in part by reading and responding to the magnetic fields around the earth, according to recent findings. The praying mantis uses ultrasonic signals to communicate, while the alligator and elephant use infrasonic ones for the same purpose. In savoring the fruits of silence and coming to value the impressions made on the mind by the qualities of the unseen, are we able to claim that there are senses to utilize and appreciate that can ripen our spirits and take us where we need to go? Is there an inner flame to life's experience that can lay waste our resistance to the ethereal and lead us beyond the solid screen of appearances so that in abandoning the dimensions of matter as the ultimate arbiter of our understanding, we can arrive once and for all at the immateriality of a sweet surrender to reality as it unfolds beyond our eyes, ears and other senses? After all, universal nature as we witness it on earth, and all the sacred signs and symbols contains therein, must go beyond and be much more than the sheer materiality they seem to represent.

The use of the sixth sense, and an appreciation of the knowledge and wisdom that comes to us through this faculty of perception, introduces the possibility of escaping from the domain of the other five senses, and allows us to redirect our emotions to those things that lie outside their domain. We have all experienced the implicit power of the sixth sense as an effective warning signal in helping us to recognize and ward off danger, without the usual suspects in the world of materiality that speak directly to the other five senses. We have all experienced that "sinking feeling", the hairs of the body standing on end, the knife-like pain within the heart or the gut wrenching feeling in the stomach that is the direct reflection of the input of the sixth sense on the body as a warning signal or the register of some deep emotion. That is why many people implicitly trust the messages of the sixth sense by virtue of its ability to preserve us from danger and keep us in good stead.

The mind thus devoid of the raw input of the senses becomes stimulated by the spiritual power that emanates from the physical objects in the world that surrounds us. Through the symbolic value implicit in every created thing, we are able to arrive, like a child, at the original simplicity and integrity that lies embedded within nature and that continually feeds us signals of a higher order of experience. If there is a sixth sense that has the power to transform thoughts and natural predilections into higher perceptions and sensibilities, then it lies outside of time and has the capacity to bring us with it into the realm of the eternal moment while even here in time, leading to experiences and encounters within the deepest aspects of ourselves that would otherwise never see the light of day. These experiences become the very threads that make up the fabric of an inner life of spirituality, forced veiled if you will to the outer world that no one will see directly, but will feel through the action of their enlightening significance. Intuitive perceptions of the mind, together with the raw spiritual instinct that is endemic to human nature, release us from the demands of the flesh and the rigidity of the physical world. They take away the burden of the senses and the heaviness of the heart with their light-hearted and otherworldly perceptions.

The experiences of the senses are like pebbles thrown into a pond, initiating hidden circles of premonition and spiritual longing that make their way through the placid lake of our inner being and disturb its serenity with feelings of wonder and awe in the face of a tantalizing mystery that unfolds in wavelets across the soul. What, then, would the experience be like of plunging headlong into the deep well within us with all of the power at the disposal of our mind and heart? Journeying from the pungent, visual, and soundful world of the formal senses to the inner ethereal world of intuition and spiritual instinct is not something that we feel entirely comfortable with. What comes naturally is that we enjoy the sights, smells and sounds for what they are in their outer compartment and not as they truly are according to their given nature and essence. In many instances, we even disbelieve the frank perceptions of the sixth sense or trust in the light of their intuited knowledge, much less rely on their frank insight and clear light guiding us through life light a flaming torch through a dark forest. Following in the footsteps of what we might learn from a hunch or a gut feeling leaves us in many instances with feelings of insecurity and unease. What would be the point of abandoning all of our allegiances to the surety of the five senses for the sake of an otherworldly experience that the intuitions of a sixth sense might provide? It would be like taking a journey into the dark interior of Africa knowing full well the hazards and risks that might lie in wait, if nothing other than a supreme solitude and eternal silence that we are apt to witness on the inward road upward toward the heavenly realms.

Beyond the efficiency and efficacy of the five senses and perhaps one step deeper into the interior lies the realm of common sense and the faculty of reason that leads us to its destination. We all know what common sense can do for us by virtue of the fact that we regularly invoke its name in reasoning ourselves through a practical dilemma. "It simply defies common sense," has become a clarion call for people when they are faced with a situation or dilemma that goes against a universal norm understood and embraced by everyone and that lies on common ground for all to see. There is in fact a sense within the human being that perceives the commonality of a thought or an impression that is the result of the collective input of the senses and upon which everyone would universally agree without question. While it is difficult to identify precisely what falls into the category of common sense, there are whole swaths of knowledge that are not self-evident and therefore do not fall under the rubric of common knowledge. There is no common sense intuition, for example, of the behavior of the universe at subatomic levels. In fact, even when we know the facts of the quantum world, we are hard put to give them meaning and/or apply that knowledge within the order of magnitude to which we are accustomed. Certain human behaviors such as good will toward humanity are generally taken as a given and therefore abide by the expectations of common sense.

As sentient beings, we have a number of instruments in the form of the five senses and a number of faculties in the form of what could be referred to as the four INs—intellect, intuition, intelligence and instinct—that help us negotiate our way through the broad labyrinth of this world with its outer maze and its inner mystery all leading toward one central point where the Supreme Treasure lay hidden. As humans we all rely on the bodily senses and human faculties in pursuit of knowledge that will enlighten us and lead us beyond the central mystery of our lives. However, the light that is properly apprehended by the senses is not the same as the light that is apprehended by the intellect and its related faculties. The sensible light of the sun drenched upon our world manifests the sensible objects within the natural order of that world, whereas the light of the mind is the true knowledge contained within our thought patterns. Sight and intellect do not actually apprehend the same light; instead each acts according to and within the limits of its own natural order. However, when those who open the eye of the intellect and whose intelligence partakes of the spiritual insight made available to it through revelation, then they are able to see with both the senses and the higher faculty of the intellect that which transcends both sense and intellect. The doctrine of divine illumination and uncreated light so prevalent in the thought and experience of the mystics down through the ages speaks of a light that belongs to the supernatural world and is altogether different from natural light that we experience here on earth within the natural order.

❧

In coming to terms with the higher, more mysterious forces that are at play within the universe and that we would be hard put to ignore at the risk of completely misunderstanding ourselves and our true nature within the scheme of things, we need to consider two key components of the human constitution that actually shed unexpected light on the true nature of knowing and perception. They are the two concepts of human consciousness and the faculty of the intellect. If we have a so-called sixth sense, then it inevitably feeds of the direct insight and intuitions of the human intellect and leads the human mind onto the broad plain of human consciousness.

Firstly, we must ask the inevitable question concerning human consciousness: What it is precisely, how it originated, what purpose it serves, and to what end it will lead humanity. Beyond the face of modern man and beyond the grasp of the modern scientific inquiry lies the enigma of man's knowledge of self, a universal mystery whose integrity as a perennial enigma has succeeded in preserving the defining quality of man's humanness from the knife-edge of man's irreverent scrutiny. Human consciousness continues to define man's humanness in ways that still elude the comprehension of the modern scientific community, much less the mass population that enjoys its benefits.

We know from the religious traditions that human consciousness represents a state of mind and a higher cognitive faculty that raises the human being above the rest of the creation. What we perhaps do not remember, by virtue of the offensive of modern science to reduce the mind to a mechanized analogue emerging out of the neurons of inorganic brain matter, is that in mirroring the Supreme Mind, human consciousness becomes a supra-sensory faculty that permits these divine qualities and attributes to become existential realities and virtues that characterize the humanness of humanity in the light of these higher spiritual attributes. We need to reflect upon and consider what the traditional mentality has known all along and what the modern mentality is not willing to admit, namely that consciousness is an artifact of the mind that irradiates the entire thinking process and links us directly to the Spirit that encompasses the cosmos.

Because of the many levels and degrees that are usually associated with the faculty of human consciousness, it could be called the spectrum of the mind whose many colors and shades actually provide the prism through which we consider the machinations of the inner self and understand the reality of the world we live in. Nothing highlights more the interaction of the world of man as microcosm and the world of the universe as macrocosm as does the mystery of consciousness. The conscious—as opposed to the animal—mind serves as a kind of witness that transcends both humanity and the world by being a quality of thought that allows experience to be viewed through a transcending mirror that witnesses the essential knowledge of God through a reflection of the self. Because of human consciousness, only the human being participates in the transcendent principle and reflects a luminous source.

That having been said, however, it must be added that consciousness lurks as an unexplained mystery in the shadow of the human form. Consciousness at the universal level recalls the color of the rainbow with its transparent hint of miracle reaching down and touching earth before disappearing again in the mist. It reflects the wisdom behind the flight of the eagle. It remembers the perfection within the design of snow crystals and the calm within the eye of the storm. It summons the beauty encompassed within the colorful forms of a butterfly wing, and the message of order and design behind the spider's web. Indeed, consciousness synthesizes a web of intricacies that encaptures all of nature and places man at the heart of it all as the one observing and listening, in search of a knowledge that lies within the cells of his being as it does beyond the outer reaches of the stars.

The depth of human consciousness, according to the early traditions of Buddhism as well as modern depth psychology, reaches back to a beginningless past with the entire universe as its basis, when consciousness became manifest as a conscious awakening to knowledge and to life. Consciousness became known to humanity when Adam first met himself in the dawn of his life. As a purely subjective being, he did not say: 'I am I'; but rather, as a subjective being capable of objectivity, he was able to say 'I am not I but He that is in me', as if he could gaze within the well of his own being and see, not himself but the Divinity that created him. In this way, the first prototype human intelligence became reflective and objectifying, as the individual consciousness re-oriented itself away from the purely physical and corporeal world toward its luminous source in the lofty realm of the Spirit. For humanity, consciousness began long ago in a far away place in the blue-white morning of the human mind. Consequently, the primordial resonance of dawn shines down through the ages of time as a crystalline quality of comprehensibility that characterizes the state of mind associated with consciousness, a brilliant clarity and a heightened presence that provides the protocol and ambiance for all human thought.

Thereafter, mankind has lived as a human entity through the power of a uniquely human consciousness. He is human man rather than hominoid man because of his consciousness of self, and he has the potential to transcend himself through a heightened consciousness that will lead back to the white light of eternity that is traditionally referred to as enlightenment. As the generations of Adam have cascaded down through the millennia, the ways and paths of the religions have whispered into the ear of the single requirement that makes people what they are as potential beings on earth and as universal beings in principle and by nature, namely the ability to see themselves as individual identities and to know themselves as a mirror reflection of a Superior Being. As such, we are beings who live 'self-consciously' in time but who exist 'supra-consciously' within eternity. As *Homo sapiens*, human intelligence is related to consciousness as time is related to eternity. As *Homo spiritualis*, to live in time is to live within the context of eternity; while to be intelligent is to take part in a consciousness that transcends the human order. There exists something in humanity whose reality belongs to an order beyond time; there exists within man the consciousness of a Reality that can envisage not only time, but also its origin in eternity and its end in transcendence.

The five senses define the elements of "this world", but remember and reflect the qualities of the "other world". Our eyes see clearly and we look directly at the reality of the world, but we remember the reality of a higher world. We hear and comprehend the voice of language and the sound of nature, but remember the voice of God. We smell the odors of life, but remember the presence of other-worldly spirits through perfume and incense. Through speech, we can articulate the narrative of our mind, and through the sense of touch we can embrace our fellow man and express the higher emotions of the spirit-world.

The ways of the spirit whisper to humanity at the dawn of day, in the final moments before sleep, in times of crisis, during moments of prayer. The ways of the spirit make themselves known when all the existential barriers have suddenly fallen away and the veils separating us from a direct perception of the true reality have been lifted. The way of the spirit reveals an unexpected awakening of human consciousness that feels like an egg has cracked open inside and poured its revelatory contents over the surface of the mind. What it is or means exactly we do not know, but it recreates the qualities of mind that we experience as fully human beings, but cannot adequately explain. The mindfulness of thought, the supreme logic of reason, the force of human will, the prescient awareness, the abiding vision of the self, and the ability to conceptualize objectively and objectify our subjective experience are all the result of this outpouring of higher consciousness. Ultimately, the faint echoes of the supreme consciousness emerge and make their presence felt, recalling primordial man and anticipating the perfect and universal man.

There is a structure associated with consciousness that we experience directly, a structure whose design is well ordered and subtle and whose power is unique and infinite. We have a knowledge within us that is encased in consciousness; it is not a thing to be studied or explained, but rather a process to be experienced. There is mystery to consciousness, on the one hand, that leaves us questioning its ultimate meaning, and there is clarity on the other hand that answers all questions and resolves all doubt. It suggests the bottomless depths of an ancient well that at the same time has the power to lead us beyond the border of our known selves. Drop a stone into this well and you listen to its descent without ever hearing its final arrival. It reaches its pinnacle of manifestation when we sense a thing without knowing it and know a thing without consciously perceiving it. The knowledge has become realized within our being and its presence is known and felt as an existential as well as an inner reality. It is an awareness that seizes the body and reaches down to the level of the cells even, and it is a mindfulness that seeps into the mind and psyche as an ethereal mist, revealing a presence that identifies who we are and a power that can change the course of our lives. Consciousness becomes the witness of all that we see and do.

The conscious mind that once drew primitive images of men and animals on a cave wall in the south of France has been an active witness to its own historical development in a vast narrative of progression and change that has taken the modern mentality to places it will never visit in person. Through instruments of our own devising, our mechanical eye gazes many millions of light years into the far reaches of the heavens and radio ears listen to the whisperings of even more remote galaxies. With the aid of sophisticated microscopes, we are able to dissect the elements of our own being and through great particle accelerators, we can (indirectly) observe the actions and consequences of the particles of sub-atomic matter. Because of our formidable, inquiring mind and the unique character of our consciousness, we have broken through the boundaries that control and limit the rest of the creation and allowed us to reach a level of speculation and thought never before envisioned in the history of humanity.

Consciousness represents a continuum and a process that cannot be denied. Memory fades; imagination falters; reason deceives; logic fails. Our intelligence can fall short of the mark and our desires and emotions change with the wind. Still, consciousness is always there—like the air to the wind, the glow to the fire, the darkness to the night, the peak to the wave and the bud to the flower. It is there because it is the necessary foundation upon which we are built, a mystery that is dark and rich and enduring, and that shares in the wisdom of the universe. The mind and its enveloping niche – consciousness – is the one intangible reality that modern science does not fully comprehend and cannot control because it has not succeeded in measuring its elusive parameters and it does not dare to deny its existential presence.[2] Perhaps therein lies the fundamental determination of the modern scientific establishment to reduce mind and consciousness to its lowest common denominator in the

2. There is some considerable irony in the fact that what actually drives the scientific inquiry forward, namely the human mind in search of the true nature of reality, slips through the fingers of curious scientists and escapes their grasp precisely because they refuse to acknowledge its metaphysical origin and supra-natural source.

ashes of purely physical matter in order to avoid the problem of coming to terms scientifically with an inviolable mystery.

The traditions do not say precisely what the mind is, or consciousness for that matter. Instead, they state what the mind—and its higher counterpart the intellect—can accomplish. The religions resort to traditional images and universal symbols to clarify the difficult but essential metaphysical concepts that everyone needs to comprehend, at least in principle. In one of the earliest traditional sources of Taoism in ancient China, Chuang Tzu, in his work entitled *The Book of Chuang Tzu*, refers to consciousness in this way: "What I mean by the expression 'having good ears' does not concern the faculty of hearing the external objects (*t'a*). It concerns only hearing one's own 'self' (*tzu*). What I mean by the expression 'having good eyes' does not concern seeing the external objects. It concerns only seeing one's own 'self'."[3] In this context, 'seeing one's own self' is a self-intuition that recalls what the Zen Buddhists call 'seeing one's [real] nature', a process that serves as a prelude and initiation to the experience of the higher consciousness that reflects not the individual self but the Supreme Self.

In the Quran, Allah is identified as the All-Seeing (*al-basir*) as well as the All-Knowing (*al-alim*), these being the two counterpoints, and the balance if you will, of a comprehensive and complete consciousness, namely a knowledge with insight and an intuitive vision based on the essential knowledge. In the words of Coomaraswamy, this 'presence of mind' is a 'point without extension' and a 'moment without duration', transcending time and place with its intuitive knowledge of the higher consciousness of God, of which man is a mirror reflection. The concept of both seeing and knowing reflects a vision of self and a knowledge of God that raises the context of consciousness above the earthly domain of humanity with its suggestion of a creative power greater than both itself and man and yet capable of being assimilated into the human being as an operative faculty of perception and self-awareness.

In traditional literature, the symbol of the "eye" has often been

---

3. Quoted in *The Unanimous Tradition*, Ranjit Fernando (ed.) (Colombo: The Sri Lanka Institute of Traditional Studies, 1991), p. 51.

employed to represent the knowing Transcendent Self that extends beyond the limited 'ego' of man and the expression of his human 'self' in reflections of the expanding reaches of the stars. The American transcendentalist R. W. Emerson touches upon this idea in his journals: "Standing on bare ground," he says, "my head bathed by the blithe air and uplifted into infinite space, all mean egotism vanishes. I become a transparent eyeball; I am nothing, I see all; the currents of the Universal Being circulate through me; I am part or parcel of God."[4] The transparent eyeball becomes an expression to denote the experience of the miracle of consciousness that sees and knows, reflecting not the contents of thought, but the channel through which the process of knowing passes. Through vision and knowledge, humans are able to take leave of their individual nothingness and transcend themselves into vehicles of the Supreme Consciousness. Through the mind's eye, the human being is able to re-enact the qualities of God within the conscious human mind.

If the universal consciousness enters the consciousness of humanity through the mind, then it takes up residence in the heart, dwelling within humanity as the "eye" of the heart (*'ayn al-qalb*) and reflected within the intellect as a perfected and universal knowledge focused through the lens of the "eye" of certainty (*'ayn al-yaqin*).[5] The Quran identifies three levels of knowledge that lead ultimately to a confirmed certainty of the truth itself. The first degree of knowledge is the knowledge of the mind, characterized in one Quranic verse as certain knowledge [*ilm al-yakin* (102:5)]. This represents the onslaught of a certainty as the result of the normal course of logic and reasoning of the mind reminiscent of what man has achieved during these times in terms of scientific discovery and technological achievement. This is balanced by the certainty that results from the *eye of certainty* or alternatively translated *the certainty of seeing* [*'ayn al-yaqin* (102:7)], in which the human being receives knowledge based on what he actually sees with his own eyes. Ultimately, the final degree of knowing results in what the Quran calls the certainty

---

4. As quoted in Loren Eiseley's *The Star Thrower*, New York, NY: Harcourt Brace & Co., 1979, p. 211.

5. In Hinduism, it recalls the frontal eye of Shiva.

of the Truth [*al haqq al yaqin* (69:51)], a certainty that lies within the "seat" of human intelligence—namely the heart of man—as "the conscious eye" and "certainty of truth" that cannot be denied.

The traditional concept of consciousness embodies within its vision the many levels and modes of expression that the word implies. This includes a state of mind that is characteristically human rather than animal, an active and reflective thinking process that negotiates its way through all thoughts and impressions, a multi-tiered and multi-angled sense of awareness, a direct consciousness of self, a defining mode of self-expression, vast realms of imagination and emotion, the force of a free will, the living presence of mind, and the power to objectify subjective experience through the internalization of an objective knowledge. Ultimately, this "spirit of mind" arrives at the abode and resting place of a higher spiritual consciousness.

As the repository and focus of true knowledge, human consciousness processes all incoming knowledge within a framework of spatial and temporal events that find their extension and meaning, not to mention their actual reality, in their trans-temporal and trans-spatial setting of higher awareness. Without such a focus, the reality of this world would seem to enjoy an independent existence in its own right and have no extension beyond its physical, spatial and temporal truth. In other words, in separating the physical from the metaphysical, the reality of the physical world would have the objectivity found in the trans-substantiating quality of physical matter amounting to a dust-to-ashes approach to the philosophy of life. Instead, the power of the human consciousness promises us more by permitting humanity to examine the contents of the mind within a framework of reality that substantiates and then transcends the three dimensional structure of this world.

As the center of objectivity, human consciousness processes incoming knowledge within a frame of reference that is independent of the reason and ratiocination of the mind. As a mode of objectivity, consciousness is "vertical" to the constant stream of thoughts, emotions, and desires that are mental, sensory, psychic and emotional and that provide the contents that the mind must evaluate and deal with. We are not just our brain and our mind in their sensorial and cognitive mode, for in claiming to 'know' things, the brain is an instrument and the mind a vehicle for knowing only the superficial aspect of a questionable reality that is externalized and peripheral with respect to our inmost being and with respect to experience that we know to be beyond the purely physical manifestation of life.

As the center of transcendence, human consciousness serves as a bridge between worlds. It processes all incoming knowledge within a framework of higher realities that are based on the intuitive knowledge of God and that are experienced as sacred sentiments and higher emotions. What commences as a mindfulness of individuality that allows the mind to be aware of itself without being limited to the boundaries of the body reaches far beyond the physical organs of the brain and the mind to become a center of irradiation that opens onto the self that knows things intuitively and with a certainty. In an external world that is full of mystery, uncertainty and doubt, our inmost being becomes our one absolute certainty whose existence and whose reality we cannot dispute or deny. Our intuitive awareness of the inner self is the very starting-point and *modus operandi* of our self-consciousness. It represents the apogee of our humanness and the watermark in the parchment of higher spiritual experience.

Behind the face of man is an inward reality and a condition of knowability that we cannot actually measure or observe, but that we know exists by virtue of our experience of its enduring presence and the power of its consequences. I have it without which this work would not be possible; you have it, otherwise you never would have gotten this far in the reading; indeed, everyone has it without which they could not function as men and women within the world since it distinguishes who men and women are as human beings within a human society. We may not know what it is precisely, but we feel its "process" working within us as a higher reality descended upon our existential world, a reality that finds its origin and source in the knowledge of God. When opened to its fullest consciousness, it will ultimately turn humanity into a human revelation and a living source of knowledge.

In the end, the power of human consciousness brings us face to face with ourselves and will lead us into the next age of humanity. Through the power of the inward 'eye' of consciousness, we can identify ourselves, not in terms of physical matter and not in a precarious alliance with a purely human reason to negotiate our way through the impenetrable mysteries of life. Only the ill-defined and unexplained presence of consciousness that lies behind the open face of humanity will give people the prescience and temerity of mind to resolve the fundamental mystery that lies at the core of the existential experience. Only the knowledge of the self will open the invisible doorway of our being, a doorway that once opened becomes the 'sun door' to a transcending and trans-luminescent world. By passing through that door, humanity will advance beyond the reality that they now know, in order to arrive at a reality that they will come to know as the true origin and ultimate source of knowledge in the Spirit of God and His abiding Presence.

Without consciousness, we would not be human; with it, we can know the Divinity and reflect His names and qualities.

Within the mind, beyond the first tier of human reasoning, lies a sun door that leads to the mysterious if not downright mystifying faculty of the intellect. This is the human faculty that draws into the inquiring mind a spiritual intuition that radiates with the perennial message of the direct knowledge of God, a sublime imperative that fuels the fire of the mind with the inner glow of the infinite and the eternal. We know enough about ourselves to realize that our intelligence and its complement the mind is the prime mover of our thinking and conscious selves; but precisely what forms its contents, how it operates, where it draws its first principles from, and what enables and sustains the vital flow of its complex and subtle activity remains a mystery without resolution, particularly to modern man who refuses to consider the sacred paradigm of knowledge that relies on the light of the first principles emanating from a divine Source to define the true nature of human intelligence. The secrets of the human mind are still not forthcoming and may never be, at least not to the modern mentality long steeped within the tradition of mathematical precision and the uncompromising exclusivity of the modern scientistic approach to understanding the world.

As we have attempted to portray throughout the course of this work, the balanced functioning of the human mind, its native intelligence, and the consciousness that provides the driving force of the human self-awakening needs inspiration and support from a source higher than itself, for the mind on its own is a *tabula rasa* of human potential waiting to be awakened and fully expressive. Left to its own devices, human intelligence is an uncertain faculty in search of a medium of true understanding, bereft of the wisdom of the ages and deprived of the spark and afterglow of an initial first knowledge.

According to the traditions of the perennial philosophy, the source of such knowledge originates within the vertical dimension whose axis intersects the horizontal plane of this world like a flaming sword from heaven and whose insight has perennially provided people the means to confidently navigate the dark realms that exist in the labyrinth of the mind. This first knowledge experienced within the mind as a mysterious and incisive light descends from above as the luminous source of intelligence that casts indiscriminate rays of light across the surface of the mind like the whirling beams of a lighthouse illuminating some stormy promontory of the mind. Every thought in the light of those celestial rays seems to have something infinite behind it. Every object seems to abide in its appointed time and place.

According to the traditional view, human intelligence exhibits a synthesizing quality that enables humans to assimilate the knowledge of all the faculties with which it is associated in order to objectify themselves to the extent that they can see their own reflection and place it within an intelligible context, that they can identify with something other than themselves, and that they can know with an objectivity and a certitude that what they conceptualize is truthful and real. The coherent interaction of the faculties that come together and are summarized by the smooth functioning of an intelligent mind produces what scientists now refer to as consilience,[6]

---

6. Even Edward Wilson, in setting the stage for the exposition of his major work entitled *Consilience*, resorts to religious terminology when speaking of his theme,

which is an explanatory power that derives part of its authority from a variety of disciplines. When the traditions accord man a central position within the cosmic frame of the hierarchy of being because of human intelligence, this is what the traditions intend to convey: Through the functioning of the human mind, through the capacity of its intelligence, and through the practical power of reason, subjective man can objectivize himself with the criteria of a principial knowledge that is in the power of his intelligence to encompass, and thus exceed the specific and individual criteria that inevitably emerge within the human mind on its own.

In Islam, however, the faculty of reason (aql),[7] while displaying qualities that go far beyond the purely rational conception of human reason as the secular norm within a purely physical reality, is considered an intermediate and mediating faculty and not the final arbiter of truth that it is considered to be *de facto* in the Western contemporary worldview. There must be another, higher faculty that can transcend the inherent limitations of the faculty of reason, a faculty that has the power to witness the truth directly, and the capacity to objectify—with a final certitude—things as they are in their reality. Aristotle has written: "One does not demonstrate principles, but one perceives directly the truth thereof." This higher faculty must have the power to place in perspective the totality of the truth. Its direct insight, and the conscious experience into the true nature of reality that accompanies such insight, could then seep down through the mind, the intelligence, and the reason to become an operative certitude guiding the life of *Homo sapiens*. Plato called this organ the *nous*, with the capacity to witness a transcending truth and grasp intuitively the first principles that underlie all of existence from the platform of certainty; Islam calls it the intellect.

in spite of his adamantly negative if not downright contemptuous, attitude toward the religious spirit. "The belief in the possibility of consilience beyond science and across the great branches of learning is not yet science. It is a metaphysical worldview, and a minority one at that, shared by only a few scientists and philosophers." p. 9.

7. The Quranic term *aql* keeps man on the straight path and prevents him from going astray. In the Quran, those who go astray are those who do not use the full extent of their reason (*wa la ya'qilun*) and thus are not able to understand what comes down to them from above.

The line of direct perception commences with the Universal Intellect, alternatively called the Universal Spirit. According to the Messenger Mohammed, upon him blessings and peace, the first thing that Allah created was the Intellect. Thereafter, the Universal Intellect began to shine forth as if through a prism into multiple 'lights' and manifests upon the earth in the form of revelation or the Word of God (*Kalimat Allah*), providing man with the objective criteria that he needs to establish his place within the Divine Design. This knowledge then passes directly into the human intellect in such a way that the content of the inspiration is direct and immediate and has descended from the highest possible source imaginable, namely the Universal Spirit (Intellect), thus making humanity capable of objectivity, not by their own resources but through the empowerment of the Universal Intellect of the Divinity in an act of consilience of the highest order of magnitude.

The revelation, which is an objective knowledge that descends from the Mind of God, allows humanity, as a primarily subjective being in this world, to become truly objective within the context of a true unity of spirit in the Reality of God. There is a direct encounter of the Divine Intellect with the human intellect, pouring into the receptive mold of the human intellect the essential contents of a divine knowledge that the intelligence needs in order to function according to its own true nature within the created world of nature and humanity, touching the human mind with a magic wand that glows with the Divine Light, the *Prima Veritas*. As a result of that encounter, the conscious human mind is forever cast within the aura of this supreme knowledge whose essence substantiates everything within its comforting embrace.

Within the collective schema of the descent of knowledge, the Universal Intellect is the metacosmic manifestation of the Supreme Unity. Revelation, as the exteriorization of the Divine Mind, is the macrocosmic manifestation of the Universal Intellect. As complement on the earthly plane, the human intellect becomes the instrument of direct perception of the essential knowledge of God, including the first principle of His Unicity and the truth of the one Reality. As such, the human intellect is not something cerebral in the manner that we understand the human mind to be, nor is it a specifically human faculty in the sense that we understand the reason to be. Instead, it represents the spiritual faculty *par excellence* with a modality of perception that rises above the human dimension of this world in a kind of spontaneous act of transcendence that arrives at a vision of the Sublime Reality. The intellect does not rely on the reflective thinking process or the cognitive principles of reason; rather it is a receptive and synthesizing faculty, capable of knowing directly and intuitively without any cognitive undertaking and therefore capable of transcending the individual person and his or her manner of thinking. Its revelatory power resolves the mystery underlying the source of true knowledge and its explanatory power conveys a feeling of overwhelming certitude that further verifies its objectivity and absolute quality.

If intelligence is the faculty of discernment and if human reason is characterized as discursive and rational, then the intellect[8] is the faculty of direct perception and of contemplation. As the transcending faculty and the instrument of synthesis, the intellect is the highest faculty of perception that is available to humanity. Human reason is the faculty of the purely individual order; pure intellect is supra-individual. Without the transcending feature of the intellect, the capacity to conceptualize metaphysical knowledge would be impossible since such rarefied knowledge lies far beyond the range of the individual domain and is of the universal order. In fact, that metaphysical knowledge is at all accessible to the human mind lies in the fact that, while we partake of the human order, we are also a manifestation of something far more mysterious and miraculous. The being that we know ourselves to be in this world is also the expression of a different quality of person by virtue of the

---

8. On the concept of the intellect, Thomas Aquinas has written: "It must be said that just as to proceed *rationally* is attributed to *natural philosophy,* because in it there is observed most greatly the mode of reason, so to proceed *intellectually* is attributed to *divine science,* because in it there is observed most of all the mode of the intellect" [*Dicendum quod sicut rationabiliter procedere attribuitur naturali philosophiae, quia in ipse observatur maxime modus rationis, ita intellectualiter procedere attribuitur divinae scientiae, eo quod in ipse observatur maxime modus intellectus. (In Boetium de Trinitate,* q. 6, art. 1, ad. 3)].

permanent and immutable principles that consecrate our deepest essence and imprint the spirit of God onto the human soul.

The intellect opens the gate of spiritual intelligence and its rarefied knowledge gains a person entry into the world of the spirit. Through the knowledge conveyed by revelation and received by the human intellect, every living person can know, with a certainty, the first origin and final end of life. The dilemma surrounding the starting-point for all cognitive processes is resolved in a higher faculty that serves as the ultimate medium between converse worlds. The point of departure for all knowledge is established in the connection of the human intellect with the knowledge of the highest Principle and is confirmed in the Pure Intellect of the Divinity. The inner life of the individual, including all the natural instincts, spiritual imagination, sacred emotions and higher consciousness, indeed the very faith humans express in the Divinity, are fully awakened and receive the direct impress of the knowledge of the Divine, thereby ushering into the higher consciousness of the mind and heart the knowledge of a complete and undivided Unity.

That *Homo sapiens* is much more than the body, more than the unique instrument of the mind, more even than the self-reflective wonder of the expansive consciousness, and that this knowledge extends far beyond the inquisitive ideas and analytical concepts deduced from the physical senses and orchestrated into a symphony of theoretical speculation, is taken as axiomatic by all the major world religions and their traditions. The power of the intellect permits people to transubstantiate their inner reality from an uncertain platform of tentative theory and speculation into an objectifying reality in order to raise themselves above the level of mundane awareness to a higher plane of consciousness and a more profound level of spiritual experience. It connects people directly with the supra-natural realities of a higher dimension, a power that passes from the human intellect to the created Intellect of Revelation and back once again into the vortex of the Universal Intellect where it lies steady and fully centered within the Godhead. It is truly the premier faculty of the borderland connecting our immediate earthly world with the world of the spirit, the faculty that objectifies the subjective reality of humanity, the faculty that fully synthesizes the great disparity of this world with the Supreme Principle of the one reality of which this world is but a pale reflection and the stuff of which shadows are made.

The spiritual faculty of intuition, as the operative agent within the human intellect of a knowledge that is inaccessible to normal intelligence and thus the five senses used in the scientific methods of investigation, takes place in full view of the mind and happens directly and unconsciously, without any seemingly formal apparatus, as a matter of spiritual instinct.[9] It enables people to perform the kind of mental tasks that they love to experience, but that they cannot account for consciously. We communicate through spoken and written words; we reason and think; we use our imagination and we dream. We plan and built cities; we farm land and feed ourselves and the world; we create literature and compose symphonies. We intuit imaginal worlds that have the power of reality and the certainty of knowledge. Mental processes are even coming to be recognized by some of the more enlightened thinkers of today as more intuitive than cognitive. Scientists themselves rely on the creative process of the mind and the imagination to initiate much of their probing, scientific inquiries. They would be loathe to admit it, but those sudden, intuitive illuminations could actually be lightning flashes of the soul that permit a person to move beyond the limits of his or her own shortcomings as a special dispensation to humanity from the Divinity.

Psychologists who research and study learning and behavior patterns are beginning to realize that people who feel and intuit their way through a challenging endeavor actually have a competitive edge over those who simply think their way through a problem in some straightforward rational manner. When they do this, they often cannot specifically account for how they arrived at their conclusion. Mathematicians do not believe that they are blindly following unconscious rules that they are incapable of knowing and believing in, nor do they think that their reasoning is based on some

9. "The infallible "instinct" of animals is a lesser "intellect," and man's intellect may be called a higher instinct." *The Essential Writings of Frithjof Schuon*, S.H. Nasr (ed.), p. 115.

arbitrary algorithmic procedure that—unknown to them—governs all of their mathematical perceptions. "What they think they are doing is basing their arguments upon what are unassailable truths— ultimately, essentially 'obvious' ones—building their chains of reasoning entirely from such truths."[10] They use their rational intelligence to make their way through complicated mathematical equations, but their intuitive intelligence could well be recognized as the dark light through which the unconscious first principles of mathematics arrive within the human mind.

Unsurprisingly, there is a vast difference between the knowledge arrived at through the efforts of human reason together with the five senses and the direct knowledge arrived at through the inimitable intuitions of the intellect. The reason of modern man investigates the knowledge of this world, while the five senses use their unique capacities to record that which they see, hear, smell, taste and touch. The sixth sense of humanity, through the faculty of the intellect, and the consciousness that makes possible a self-reflective mode of analysis and synthesis, participates in the knowledge of the metaphysical world of the spirit. Both forms of knowledge pass through the human mind and are filtered through human intelligence as key components to the practical functioning of people in dealing with this world. Intuitive intelligence needs the practicality of the reason to cope with the existentialities of this world, whereas the faculty of human reason needs the light of the intellect to make the essential knowledge shine forth as a guiding star in the dark firmament of the mind.

When our intelligence is cut off from its luminous source, our knowledge, our judgment, our insight and indeed our sense of discernment will be seriously diminished during the course of life. Under these conditions, there is no way that these faculties can function to their fullest capacity, in accordance with what is true to human nature. Sadly, the modern mentality does not accord the intellect its true value as a spiritual faculty capable of direct knowledge of God. Although modern individuals still have an intellect,

10. Roger Penrose, *Shadows of the Mind: A Search for the Missing Science of Consciousness* (Oxford: Oxford University Press, 1996), p. 127.

they do not know they have it. Therefore, they have nothing to effectively counterbalance the tenebrous inclination of the human mind to roam aimlessly through the dark and labyrinthine corridors of idle theory and pure speculation in search of the solid ground of a certainty that only the reality of the Spirit can provide.

People today have the gift of intelligence and they enjoy its multitudinous fruits, of this there is no doubt. In today's modern world, however, we falter and hesitate in our definition of terms: What is the mind, what defines consciousness, what is the stuff of intelligence and where will our intelligence lead us? We have the duty to ask ourselves not only whether consciousness, mind, and intelligence is enough to serve our needs, but also to what end? Opinions differ on the key fundamentals that shape the contemporary worldview and yet the goal seems to be the attainment of a knowledge that does justice to human intelligence: to be intelligent, to live intelligently, and to connect with the Supreme Intelligence with the golden thread of faith and desire. We need to free ourselves from an undue reliance on all speculative and ego-serving ideas whose only source is the human mind blundering on its own without the aid of Heaven. We need to turn away from the downward drift of human pride and pretension and submit ourselves to that which surpasses us. We need to surrender to the divine paradigm of knowledge and the source of all wisdom that alone has the power to illuminate the mind and lift up the heart.

A final thought leads us to reaffirm that behind the natural workings of the human intelligence lies a supra-natural faculty, a third eye if you will or a sixth sense, whose luminosity shines down on the mind—with all of its faculties of knowing and perception—like rays of light penetrating woodland trees to reach the forest floor. If reason is in principle a *tabula rasa* whose innocent void awaits a true knowledge that will awaken a world, then human intelligence is a playing field awaiting the illuminative rays of the intellect, the intuitive and supra-rational faculty within the kingdom of humanity, around which are gathered the ministers of state in the form of the noble faculties of reason, intelligence, imagination, and the higher emotions acting in unison with the five senses of seeing, hearing, smelling, tasting and touching. They all contribute to the qualitative expression of the human species; they all make humans what they truly are. It is only because intelligence is touched by the light of the intellect that individuals can reflect upon their human condition and say: I am a thinking creature created as a reflected image of the Supreme Intelligence; I am a shadow of the Divine Light; I am a soul whose ground reflects the luminous rays of the Divine Spirit; I am a subjective entity capable of objectivity because the Absolute has taken up residence within the cave of my heart as the living principle of my being.

In the end, our approach to the spiritual realities and the achievement of some measure of proximity to the Divine Throne is like roaming under the open, free space of the night sky, knowing that above the earth lies a configuration of stars that will always remain incomprehensible to the mind, yet strangely familiar to the soul. We need to go through life partaking not only of the pleasures that the five senses have to offer, but also basking in the light of a knowledge that comes to us either directly through sight, sound, smell, taste and touch, or indirectly through the inner senses and faculties of our intellect, intuition, intelligence and spiritual instincts. We need to journey across the great plain of our lives steeped in the mystery of every created thing, from the grand edifice of the universe to the intricacies of the spider's web, as we drift like butterflies in search of nectar over the landscape of human experience.

There are textures to the world and patterns in life that have their counterpart in celestial realities, if only we could open the door to the inner senses of perception. We go through life in terror of the unknown mystery that challenges our waking moments, when all the while we only needed to see the outstretched branches of the tree reaching heavenward in order to recognize its benevolent smile and yearning for the Divinity. Then the vastness of eternity could be taken in through the blink of an eye and the expanse of infinitude could be reduced to a single first step as we make our way on that final journey into the interior of the self.

> "I said to the almond tree,
> 'Sister, speak to me of God.'
> And the almond tree blossomed."
> (Nikos Kazantzakis, St. Francis)

EPILOGUE:
A CRACK IN THE WALL

God's joy moves from unmarked box to unmarked box,
From cell to cell. As rainwater, down into flowerbed.
As roses, up from ground.
Now it looks like a place of rice and fish,
Now a cliff covered with vines,
Now a horse being saddled.
It hides within these,
Till one day it cracks them open. (Rumi)[1]

We have explored throughout this work the inside dimension of the five senses and the untold story of their value as instruments of enlightenment and not just as vehicles of verification of the physical reality of the natural world. One final question needs asking by way of epilogue: Is there a crack in the wall of modern science, a crack so miniscule that we are lulled into believing that we can live along its fault line in comparative safety without upsetting the adamantine certitude of the modern scientific worldview?

In today's world, science strives for objectivity through the use of the five human senses. We are able to verify to the satisfaction of the rational mind what the senses tell us in terms of size, shape, and color. What we cannot verify directly, we then verify indirectly through machines that record activity of the atomic and quantum worlds when the direct vision of the eyes fails to witness and record what takes place at the sub-atomic level. As such, scientists boast that the theories and discoveries of modern science make the physical reality well within our reach, either through the instruments of

1. *Open Secret: Versions of Rumi*, tr. John Mayne and Coleman Barks (Putney, VT: Threshold Books, 1984), p. xiii.

the senses or through the pursuit of an instrumental science that has prodigiously extended its grasp over physical reality. We can now boast that having been blind for millennia, we can now see— literally. We have learned, for example, that visible light is not the only illuminating energy within the universe. It is actually an infinitesimal spec of electro-magnetic radiation comprising wavelengths of 400 to 700 nanometers (billionths of a meter), creating radiation that rains continuously down upon our bodies. Before we had the luxury of modern-day instruments to measure such activity, we were oblivious to its existence.

When we were once deaf; now everything is available to our ears through the use of rarefied instruments that mock the skills of the natural senses. Humans have a natural auditory range from 20 to 20,000 Hz per second. We now know that flying bats broadcast ultrasonic pulses into the night air above that range and listen for echoes to locate moths and other insects on the wing. Before the 1950s, zoologists were unaware of this nocturnal contest. Now, with receivers, transformers and night-time photography, they can follow every squeak and aerial performance of cat and mouse between predator and prey with the ease of special equipment.

The descent into *minutissima* in the search for the ultimate building blocks of matter and life seems to be the driving mania of the modern scientific establishment. This search for the ultimate particle has been aided through steady advances in the resolving power of microscopes, in response to the ultimate human craving to see the reality with the human eye. The most powerful modern instruments developed in the 80s are the scanning-tunneling microscope and the atomic force microscope which provides an almost literal view of atoms bonded into molecules and the DNA double helix. Atomic-level imaging is the end product of three centuries of technological innovation in search of direct observation with the "aided eye". Microscopy began with the primitive optical instruments of Anton van Leeuwenhoek, which in the late 1600s revealed bacteria and other objects a hundred times smaller than the resolution of the human eye. It has arrived at methods for showing objects a million times smaller, resulting now in the fast developing science of nanotechnology.

We have discovered that solid matter as the foundation that bears the weight of the entire fabric of modern science is actually empty space. The solidity of iron is actually 99.9999999999 percept vacuous space made to feel solid by ethereal force fields that, technically speaking, have no material reality. Quantum physics has now revealed that what we perceive as a particle may also be a wave and vise versa, leading to conjecture that, on the physical plain, there is no fixed or tangible reality at all, a truth that the religions have proclaimed all along. Consider, for example, the sound of music. The waves of sound that enter my eardrum in a beautifully complex path become electrical pulses that are chemically stored in the cortex of my brain. But how do I hear the sound and how does its implicit beauty become apparent and appreciated? Where is the vision or the smell? Which of those formerly inert atoms of carbon, hydrogen, nitrogen, and oxygen in my head have become so clever that they can produce a thought or reconstitute an image? How sense data are recalled and replayed into sentience remains an enigmatic mystery to modern science without an impending solution in sight. Where is the passageway that leads from brain to mind to consciousness?

We live within a certain frame of reference that is becoming increasingly enigmatic, in spite of the tremendous advancements of science and their technological achievements. It is as if in reducing the physical components of life to their most common denominator we are releasing, as though through a crack in the wall of speculation, the sentient wisdom of life that is not apparent in the purely physical form of those structures. We know that atoms make up the quantum structure of brains as they do all other physical realities, and neurons of the brain connect to produce a mind that creates thoughts that lead ultimately to human desires; but what is the true relationship between a human desire and the senses that crave their physical satisfaction. "Nothing is hidden, neither an atom, but that it is written." (10:61)

We have embarked on a solitary voyage into the unknown world of the inner life of the senses, a story that needed to be told to modern-day seekers who are having trouble reading between the lines of the phenomenal world, who would like to believe in a higher reality, but find it difficult in this overwhelming modern and secular society, who see cracks in the wall but do not discern the secret messages within their opening. We live within the continuum of time and within the world of the senses. We see, we hear, and we do all those other things that the senses record for us as the truth of the matter, and we walk away thinking that we have arrived at the resolution to the mystery of existence and the perennial challenge of the human condition. We put our faith in "this world", when one of the sayings of the Prophet Mohammed encourages the faithful to live for the unseen world. We live in this world as if we will live forever, whereas we should live for the next world as if we will enter it tomorrow.

If that was all there was to it, then perhaps we would be justified in thinking, as we do today, that we live and we die and the world passes on spinning like a top until the law of thermodynamics has the final word and the drama of the great human narrative will come to an end. What would our response be, however, if we noticed a crack in the continuum of time to reveal for a split second the realm of eternity surrounding the continuum of time in the same way that outer space surrounds the earth and its solar system; what would we think if saw a crack in the universe itself, revealing not a parallel universe as modern science lead us to believe, but an expanse of infinity outside the box of the universe. We rely once again on the mystic poet Rumi to answer our question, quoted at the beginning of this epilogue. Could it be that God's joy hides within the brightness of the sun and the depths of the oceans, as the husk within the kernel or the egg within the shell, until one day these things crack open to reveal what the great world religions have proclaimed all along?

Rumi lends us an insight that might help us see the light of day once more and steer us toward the direction we are destined for. "I'm crying, my tears tell me that much." Yes indeed, here are my tears; but do I know why I am crying? Let us look at the evidence that the senses reveal in order to understand their implicit wisdom, rather than accepting answers that bear no relation to the question. The mist of dawn creeps over the horizon with the coming day holding secrets that we cannot afford to ignore. Birds' voices sing a melody whose joy we need to listen to. The moody colors in the garden and the exquisite smell of flowers sing of immortality through color and form. The greatest wonder is that the mystery and insight that linger behind all the created forms of nature have the capacity to ease our confusion and wipe clean our sorrows and insecurities, if only we had our vision, hearing, smell, and sense of taste and touch attuned to the wisdom of their inner messages.

> *See, where thou nothing seest;*
> *Go, where thou canst not go;*
> *Hear, where there is no sound;*
> *Then where God speaks art thou.*[2]

In the Gospels, Jesus has said, on the one hand, "I shall give you what no eye has seen and what no ear has heard and what no hand has touched and what has never occurred to the human mind." (1 Clem 38:8) It is almost as if he were referring to the crack in the wall of the senses I referred to earlier, that there are wonders to behold and sounds to be listened to that are not of our reckoning. He has also said, on the other hand, "When you fashion an eye in place of an eye, and a hand in place of a hand, and a foot in place of a foot, and a likeness in place of a likeness, then you will enter the Kingdom."[3] In other words, there is an inner eye that sees, an inner hand that produces good works, and an inner foot that will take us where we need to go, so long as we "see through the crack" as it were, to find ourselves on the other side. Once we have gained access, the joy of the universe will be there to behold. "You will never enjoy the world aright till the sea itself floweth in your veins, till you are clothed with the heavens and crowned with the stars, and perceive yourself to be the sole heir of the whole world. Till you can sing and rejoice and delight in God, as misers do in gold, as Kings in scepters, you never will enjoy the world. Till your spirit fillet the whole world, and the stars are your jewels; til you are as familiar with the way of God in all ages as with your walk and table; till you are

---

2. Angelus Silesius, *The Cherubinic Wanderer*, written under the pen name of "The Silesian Angel", *Not of this World* (Bloomington, IN: World Wisdom Books, 2003), p. 259

3. Ibid., p. 160.

intimately acquainted with that shady nothing out of which the world was made; till you love men so as to desire their happiness, with a thirst equal to the zeal of your own; till you delight in God for being good to all: you will never enjoy the world."[4]

Locked within the five senses lies the secret of some final emotion that begins to emerge every time we reach beyond ourselves and experience the world with the inner senses, whether it be through our body, mind or soul. We go through life touching surfaces, exploring possibilities and promises, probing depths within the well of the world for a deeper meaning and final emotion that will lift us out of ourselves and set us down on some mountain peak where we can watch the clouds pass by. We use our cognitive mind to witness within the mirror of the natural order the supra-natural world expressive of the metaphysical reality. The possibility of happiness that we cherish throughout our lives, and that we pursue with rigor through the benedictions of the five senses, is a happiness that we wish to see and feel and taste with an intensity so great that a sense of transcendence shines through the cracks, so that the senses offer up to us not only a paradise of sensations, but the promise of an enduring reality that lies far beyond their reach.

As votive candles in the darkness of our lives, the senses contain a promise that we cannot afford to ignore, because they lead to that final emotion that we cannot afford to live without, namely the love of God as the one true Beloved and the one true Reality. What begins as a leap of faith in Islam as a way of resolving the fundamental mystery of life, eventually transforms into a love of God that no one can take away. Then, all our experiences and all the years of our lives can unfold in one sweet unraveling, leaving behind the core of love's essence as witness to all that we have accomplished.

> Love makes dead bread into soul,
> Love makes the mortal soul immortal.
> (Rumi)

---

4. Ibid., p. 129.